Enjoy,

C. Mor

TESTOSTERONE

STRONG ENOUGH FOR A MAN, MADE FOR A *Woman*

TESTOSTERONE

STRONG ENOUGH FOR A MAN, MADE FOR A *Woman*

PS: WE HAD IT WRONG

DR. CHARLES MOK

ForbesBooks

Published by ForbesBooks, Charleston, South Carolina.
Member of Advantage Media Group.

ForbesBooks is a registered trademark, and the ForbesBooks colophon is a trademark of Forbes Media, LLC.

Printed in the United States of America.

ISBN: 978-0-99836-550-3
LCCN: 2016960998

10 9 8 7 6 5 4 3 2

Cover design by Katie Biondo.

This publication is designed to provide accurate and authoritative information in regard to the subject matter covered. It is sold with the understanding that the publisher is not engaged in rendering legal, accounting, or other professional services. If legal advice or other expert assistance is required, the services of a competent professional person should be sought.

Advantage Media Group is proud to be a part of the Tree Neutral® program. Tree Neutral offsets the number of trees consumed in the production and printing of this book by taking proactive steps such as planting trees in direct proportion to the number of trees used to print books. To learn more about Tree Neutral, please visit **www.treeneutral.com.**

Since 1917, the Forbes mission has remained constant. Global Champions of Entrepreneurial Capitalism. ForbesBooks exists to further that aim by bringing the Stories, Passion, and Knowledge of top thought leaders to the forefront. ForbesBooks brings you The Best in Business. To be considered for publication, please visit **www.forbesbooks.com**

TABLE OF CONTENTS

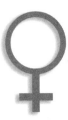

Acknowledgments

I would like to thank the people who inspired or helped me write this book. This is by no means a complete list but are notable mentions.

My journey into the research for a modern approach to testosterone for women was inspired by Susan Burg. She was having problems with traditional natural hormone replacement, as we knew it at the time. With fresh eyes, I started looking into the advances in this field of medicine.

To Rebecca L. Glaser, MD, FACS, a breast cancer surgeon who, in my opinion, has done the most breakthrough work on what we will be talking about in much of this book—primarily replacing testosterone, instead of estrogen, for women as they age.

To Mary Carr, Master's in Library Science at McLaren Macomb Medical Center, for responding so quickly and politely to my seemingly never-ending request for original research articles.

To Mary Scott, our marketing director, who was the liaison with our editors and publisher.

And to my wife, Natalie, who tolerated the constant mess I had around my den, living room, and sitting room, cluttered with countless medical journals I assembled to better tell this story.

Foreword

Hormones that are chemically identical to human (CIH) have been available for decades. Their safety and effectiveness for health, disease prevention, and cure have now been confirmed by thousands of studies. Yet they are not universally used. Hormone status should be considered during most adult health care, but it isn't. Physicians who are up-to-date should use hormones as medication. It has been proven to prolong disease-free life and treats many of the common diseases of the elderly, including the biggest killers: heart disease, diabetes, some cancers, and probably some neurological diseases.

The non-CIH hormones are vastly inferior and should be banned. These include Premarin®, which is horse-urine manufactured (equine) estrogen, and Provera®, a chemical related to progesterone. These two cause health problems in many studies. (Prem-pro® and other brands are the same thing.) Yet they are still being actively marketed, totaling billions of dollars in revenues.

The goal is to raise hormone blood levels in patients to roughly match a younger person's. This produces improved health, which can be felt by the patient and measured by various tests. However, claims about exact standards for desirable blood levels are false. No clear standards exist. And judging "proper" blood level against "normal aging" blood levels—which are low—is wrong. Generally, what feels best is a good guide to doses. Physicians are trained with treatment of symptoms, yet often think more of blood levels.

The "hormone-as-therapy" scientific literature is huge. Dr. Mok has spent decades working with these issues and this science and has massive clinical experience. He is one of the most respected and experienced clinicians in the country for womens' health and cosmetic medicine. This book has Dr. Mok's conclusions.

The hormone standard of care is broken. Dr. Mok will explain why.

—Robert Yoho, MD
Pasadena, California

PS: This book has all this plus two fortune cookies (spoiler alert). There is information about testosterone pellets. It turns out that testosterone—which is metabolized into other hormones—can be used as a sole agent to reduce breast cancer and treat hormone deficiency. And there's fascinating information about the brave new world of how the bacteria in your colon influence your chances of obesity and how Dr. Mok is studying cures.

Introduction

Breast cancer and other risks may increase with commonly used hormone replacement therapy (HRT). You've no doubt heard this information many times before, as have millions of other women. But this is a myth that has been perpetuated for years by the research community, the medical community, and the media, and it has created a fear of HRT that has kept women from living long, healthy, and productive lives.

The reality is that there are specific drugs that were designed to replace hormones that, in a certain setting, increase certain diseases. But the generalization that hormone replacement with actual human hormones is linked to an increase in diseases is absolutely false.

The fear stems from large clinical trials that evaluated the safety of a common menopause hormone substitution therapy combining Premarin and Provera, two synthetic drugs manufactured by a large pharmaceutical company that were intended to treat symptoms of menopause. For two decades, these synthetic hormones were not only the top prescribed treatments for women in the United States experiencing menopause; they were also the most commonly pre-scribed drugs in America.

At the onset of menopause symptoms—the period known as *peri-menopause*—the ovaries are still functioning, but they're beginning to run out of eggs, and ovarian estrogen production is becoming erratic. Premarin and Provera were designed to copy estrogen (Premarin) and progesterone (Provera) and to be used to replace these declining hormones.

Premarin is a conjugated equine estrogen (CEE)—or as I call it, "horse estrogen." It is a copy of the estrogen makeup of a five-year-old, pregnant mare. Horses have a large variety of estrogens that are similar in some ways to humans; however, there are only three types of human estrogen: estrone, estriol, and estradiol. Provera is a synthetic progestin designed to mimic the effect of naturally occurring progesterone and protect the uterus against stimulation by Premarin.

The Change—in HRT and in My Career

HRT has undergone a dramatic transformation. Decades ago, only women with significant symptoms were treated with HRT. In the 1980s, 1990s, and early 2000s, hormone replacement became widespread for women entering menopause, regardless of the severity of their symptoms. The transition stemmed from several studies that showed HRT to be beneficial in preventing cardiac disease and other health issues in menopausal women.

The biggest change came shortly after the Women's Health Initiative (WHI) released its findings in the early 2000s. The WHI was composed of multiple clinical trials that observed thousands of menopausal women to assess the effects of horse estrogen and synthetic progestin on them. The results showed an increase in breast cancer and other health risks in women taking horse estrogen and synthetic progestin. Women taking horse estrogen alone (because they had no uterus due to a prior hysterectomy) did not have an increase of breast cancer risk.

The WHI trial results were the first widely accepted evidence calling into question the practice of using synthetic hormones routinely in women. Confusion over the results of the trials led to a widespread reduction of the use of HRT to manage the symptoms of menopause. There was widespread belief that HRT in and of itself was the culprit; no distinction was made between the synthetic and natural hormone forms of the treatments at the time. There were other substantial flaws in the original interpretation of the results that I will talk about in the chapters ahead.

The WHI study confusion was instrumental in influencing me to change my career.

Prior to the release of the WHI findings, I was a doctor working in the emergency and trauma center at a teaching hospital. It was a great job. As vice chairman of the department, part of my job was to train residents to become specialists. I also trained them to critically review medical literature in a process we called the "Journal Club." I would select a topic of medical research, and we would read the associated studies. Then we took turns presenting the studies, which gave us the opportunity to review them for flaws. We also used the studies to determine changes in the way we practiced medicine.

During my ten-plus years at the trauma center, I helped patients who had health emergencies that were frequently preventable. For instance, I'd treat a heart attack patient with clot-busting drugs followed by an angioplasty, in which a wire was inserted into the blood vessel to stretch it open so blood could flow again. My interaction with these seriously ill or injured patients was fairly brief; I'd work with other specialists to provide the patient the appropriate care and admit them to the hospital.

After so many years of seeing the end result of poor lifestyle choices, I decided to move my career into more of a preventive role. I spent countless hours retraining myself in preventive health, and I started a practice aimed at filling the void between traditional primary care and the management of the results of disease.

A New Direction

Before and since the release of the WHI findings, there have been countless studies showing how menopause symptom relief can be achieved safely using what's known as *natural hormone replacement*. Natural hormones are nothing new. These are exact copies of human hormones and have been used in the United States and around the world for years.

The most commonly prescribed natural hormones are estradiol (which is sometimes mixed with another natural estrogen called *estriol* or *BiEst*) and natural progesterone. These can be taken by mouth or applied to the skin. Using the human versions of progesterone and estrogen instead of horse-based estrogen and synthetic progestin, numerous studies have shown not only quality-of-life improvements but also decreased disease and mortality rates.

In addition to menopausal relief and reducing the risks associated with synthetic hormones, natural hormones also offer the following benefits:

- They do not appear to increase risk of breast cancer, and may protect against breast cancer.
- They are beneficial to the heart, brain, circulatory system, and skin.
- They lead to a greater than 70 percent reduction in fatal heart attacks if taken long term.
- They even protect against belly fat.

Now for the Real News

In addition to the two hormones that most doctors think of as the predominant female hormones—estrogen and progesterone—there's a third major sex hormone that comprises what I call the "Big Three": testosterone.

Now, you might think of testosterone as a male hormone. Yes, men have more testosterone than women. But w*omen have five to twenty times as much testosterone as estrogen.* This news can be confusing, even for many doctors.

• •

Estrogen and testosterone are listed as different units of measurement on lab reports. While total estrogen is reported in picograms per milliliter (pg/ml), total testosterone is reported in nanograms per deciliter (ng/dl), with picograms or nanograms measuring mass, while milliliters and deciliters measure volume. Ten pg/ml equals one ng/dl.

Consider this example of an actual lab test on a fifty-two-year-old female.
Testosterone: 62 ng/dl
Estradiol: 30 pg/ml

To make the units the same
Testosterone 620 pg/ml and estradiol 30 pg/ml
or
Testosterone 62 ng/dl and estradiol 0.3 ng/dl
In both cases, it is 20:1.

• •

So if you're a woman supplementing hormones, do you need to add testosterone to the list? Yes!

Testosterone reduces the symptoms of menopause and has no major adverse side effects.

Testosterone improves the following:

- hot flashes
- sweating
- sleep problems
- moodiness
- irritability/anxiety
- fatigue
- joint and muscle pain
- bladder symptoms
- sexual desire, activity, and satisfaction
- thickness and fullness of scalp hair
- bone density
- memory loss
- vaginal dryness

More importantly, when added to any other HRT, testosterone significantly reduces your risk of breast cancer and heart disease.

That's a message worth repeating: *Testosterone reduces your chances of breast cancer and heart disease whether or not you are on any form of HRT.* There is even evidence that testosterone can be safely used to reduce all symptoms of menopause in women who have had breast cancer without putting them in harm's way. Testosterone also appears to protect against recurrence of breast cancer. In fact, there is evidence that testosterone can shrink the size of an existing breast cancer tumor. Low testosterone in women is a very strong predictor of the eventual development of heart disease, and normal or elevated testosterone is cardioprotective. In fact, low testosterone in women is a more accurate predictor of heart disease than cholesterol or other lipids, which are the standard metrics currently used to measure risk.

A Look Ahead

In the following chapters, I'll discuss studies that demonstrate that natural hormone replacement is integral to good health and that, along with diet and exercise, it can help prevent disease.

I will explain how the drugs that have traditionally been used to treat menopause put women at a slight increased risk of breast cancer and other health risks, such as heart disease and blood clots.

I'll review how using exact copies of a woman's natural hormones does not cause an increased risk of breast cancer or other diseases but in fact reduce risks.

I'll also discuss how adding a third, virtually neglected hormone—testosterone—to the mix actually *reduces the incidence of breast cancer*. If used alone, this forgotten hormone reduces risk of breast cancer by about 50 to 75 percent in addition to relieving virtually all symptoms of menopause with no adverse effects in clinical studies.

I will review how natural hormone replacement is not only cardioprotective but, when taken long term, actually reduces the incidence of fatal heart attacks by over 70 percent, unlike synthetic hormone drugs, which have been linked to heart disease. I will also discuss how natural hormone replacement doubles cardiac performance in women with preexisting heart disease.

The message I want to get out to the community, and what triggered me to write this book, is that the medical community got it wrong decades ago, and today there is an exciting alternative.

That alternative has helped me grow from a solo practice in a shared office space (aided only by my assistant, Crystal, who still works with me and has grown into a surgical technician) to a practice of five large offices and more than two hundred employees offering multiple health services. Our practice is in multiple cities in metro Detroit and is part of a parent company, Allure Medical Spa.

Instead of the decades-old, universally accepted practice of administering synthetic drugs through a suboptimal delivery system, we offer dramatically superior hormone replacement.

It has been an exciting journey for me, going from treating existing diseases to helping people prevent disease in the first place. In the chapters ahead, I'm going to make my case for taking this journey using several clinical studies. I want to show you scientific proof of why I'm such an advocate for natural hormone replacement.

If you are a woman seeking relief from the symptoms of menopause or perimenopause and also want to improve your overall health, HRT is absolutely your best choice. With natural—not synthetic—hormones, the risk of breast cancer, obesity, osteoporosis, and heart disease can be reduced while making you healthier and feel better. I want you to see how women who are treated with the most modern, natural, physiologically ideal hormones enjoy better sex lives, more energy, better hair, better skin, healthier hearts, more ideal weight, and likely longer lives.

Chapter 1

MENOPAUSE: A SCIENTIFIC OVERVIEW

What does it mean to "age gracefully"? As a woman, it means you're doing all you can to avoid obesity, hair loss, saggy skin, decreased sexuality, heart disease, breast cancer, diabetes, and Alzheimer's. In short, it means you're trying to look good and feel good while avoiding disease—all in an effort to ultimately delay death.

The practice of treating menopause and extending the period of maximum health has its detractors, their logic being that aging and menopause are normal parts of life, and nature should be allowed to take its course. But let's face it: numerous other diseases occur as a woman ages, and they occur at a much higher frequency when hormones decline with menopause. Menopause is a period of accelerated aging for most women. Avoiding treatment for menopause because it is a part of "normal" aging is as absurd as avoiding treatment for hypertension or diabetes, which are also associated with "normal" aging.

If you're a woman experiencing any of the symptoms of peri-menopause or menopause, it probably seems like you're waging an uphill battle. Even if you're making healthy lifestyle choices, such as better diet, regular exercise, learning and doing, being open-minded and generous, and positively influencing your family and community, you still have to manage the symptoms of your aging body and mind.

Menopause is defined as that period of time after you've experienced no menstrual cycles for one year or after you've undergone the surgical removal of the ovaries. Although that is the definition of menopause, it can be insidious and can occur quite fast for women, while others may be in and out of menopause symptoms for years before true menopause. Though the ovaries are commonly believed to be the primary source of estrogen, it can also be made in other cells, including those in the adrenal glands, the liver, fat, and the brain. In fact, most organs can likely synthesize estrogen. In the human body, estrogen actually starts out as cholesterol, which is then converted into various androgens (including testosterone). The conversion process is conducted through an adrenal enzyme known as *aromatase*.

At the onset of menopause symptoms—the period known as *perimenopause*—the ovaries are still functioning, but they're beginning to run out of eggs, and ovarian estrogen production is starting to be erratic. This is when most women should begin thinking about replacing their missing hormone production.

Today, we have solidly established HRT solutions for women experiencing perimenopause or menopause. And there's a bonus—the same HRT solutions that can make you feel and look better can also save your life.

Yes, menopause is just part of aging, but there's nothing wrong with a woman wanting the second half of her life to be as fulfilling as the first. Just as there are treatments for hypertension and other age-related diseases and conditions, there is viable treatment today for the symptoms of menopause.

HRT's time has come, but its road has been a long one that is still strewn with people who would have you believe otherwise. I've written this book to help clear the air by discussing the scientific studies that have created milestones—and in some cases hurdles—along the way.

It's All About the Impact

Centuries ago, doctors learned in more or less an apprentice system, relying heavily on their trainers, their own experiences, or the experience of peers. Following the apprentice system came the scientific method, where doctors went beyond what they thought was best to searching for actual proof based on research. Textbooks were created based on summaries of the contemporaneous literature.

In the past few decades, health care has moved more toward what's known as *evidence-based medicine* because we've developed new information, technologies, cures, and scientific proof at a pace that greatly exceeds the old paradigms of creating textbooks or relying on information being handed down from the previous generation. Doctors who keep up with science rely on peer-reviewed journals to improve their knowledge and understanding of the best patient care.

In the chapters ahead, I'm going to explain the impact that we, as physicians and scientists, have on the health-care landscape amid a constant barrage of new drugs and treatments. All of these new entries into the market can potentially affect health care, but many of them can also have unintended consequences or may only work as well as random chance. That's why research is so critical.

While discoveries can come from laboratories in universities and pharmaceutical companies, they also frequently come from individual (or groups of) health-care practitioners. A doctor specializing in a particular condition may be exposed to unrelated information that benefits one of his or her patients. That provider may study the new information, talk to colleagues, and make an assumption of the potential of a benefit for his or her patient. At that point, there is no proof, but the provider's knowledge and expertise allows him or her to try the new treatment after assessing the risk and benefit ratio. If the result is a benefit, the provider may continue the treatment. Eventually, a clinical study may be organized to explore whether the treatment offers a true benefit, whether it is safe, or whether the results represent random chance. Later, larger studies may be conducted to verify the original study's results. Eventually, if the studies are positive, a new drug is released or a new procedure is adopted.

How the Practice of Medicine Adapts

In practice, shifts in the way health care is delivered often occur in small steps. Let me explain by using the example of how emergent heart attacks are handled, a procedure that has changed dramatically over the years.

Throughout my medical school and early residency years, when a patient presented with a heart attack, diagnosis began with an electrocardiogram (EKG) and blood tests. The blood tests weren't very accurate, but they were helpful when the EKG didn't provide enough information. After the patient was admitted, we'd administer nitroglycerin, oxygen, and blood thinners, and we'd hope that the patient's symptoms would subside. In a little over 10 percent of the cases, a heart attack ultimately led to death—either the heart attack continued and the patient developed a fatal, abnormal heartbeat, or the heart would weaken, leading to congestive heart failure.

In those instances where the symptoms subsided and the patient survived, the patient might ultimately receive a heart catheterization—an insertion of a tube to help diagnose or treat the problem. If significant disease was present, the patient might receive a heart bypass. Angioplasty—the insertion of a balloon in a blood vessel or artery to widen it—was a new procedure at the time as an alternative to a bypass.

In the middle of my residency, scientists discovered a series of powerful clot-busting drugs that could stop a heart attack in its early stages. They were fairly remarkable, reducing deaths by about 30 percent. But the drugs came with a risk: a small number of people would develop fatal bleeding. So experiments were designed to determine if the drug was worth the risk. It turned out that even considering the potentially severe side effects, we needed to use the clot-busting drugs in all eligible heart attack victims—and the quicker, the better.

That discovery led to a major paradigm shift. No longer did we just wait to see what happened with a heart attack; now we could have an impact on survivability. But doctors were reluctant to use these new clot-busting drugs, even though they saved lives and reduced deaths by 30 percent.

It took a major public relations blitz and forceful pressure to get doctors to convert from "wait and see" to "treat with risky medication and save lives." At the time, information moved fairly slowly, and doctors were resistant to acknowledge that they could be doing something better for their patients rather than "doing what we have always done."

In the hospital where I worked, that transition took a series of meetings between the heart doctors, surgeons, and emergency doctors. There was much debate before we came to an agreement on the best course of action. I recall that one cardiologist even wanted to wait "until it is in the textbooks," which of course takes years.

It took some time, but eventually the clot-busting drugs became the standard of care.

Very shortly after the clot-busting drugs turned management of heart attacks upside down, evidence came to the forefront that angioplasties, which could be performed without major surgery, should be done immediately rather than after waiting weeks. The studies showed that the angioplasty procedure was better and safer than clot-busting drugs and was of course far superior to the "wait and see" approach just a decade earlier.

Again, doctors resisted and made excuses for why they shouldn't have to perform a potentially lifesaving procedure in the middle of the night, which is when most heart attacks occur. Part of their concern was the simple fear of performing what is always a relatively risky procedure. But the evidence of angioplasty survival rates was so overwhelming that, again, champions rallied at each hospital to force the issue.

The changes in treatment for heart attacks are just one example that shows the impact we providers have on health care. Today, with information such as scientific papers and studies instantly available via the Internet, patients can be more informed about their health-care options than ever before. In the past, such information was only available through subscriptions to medical journals delivered to doctors' homes or shelved in the hospital library. In fact, earlier in my career as a physician, I reviewed about a dozen medical journals a month, each containing numerous studies. Today, with an online subscription, I have virtually unlimited access to all the scientific literature that is published—literature that is aimed at physicians such as myself and is not intended for the general public.

Similarly, significant changes have occurred in heart attack management, progressing from "wait and see" to clot-busting drugs to angioplasty. That doesn't mean early methods were wrong; it just means that was all we knew. But as new information has presented itself, accepting and acting on it has led to saving countless lives.

While menopause symptoms may seem less dire than a heart attack, they are no less important to the millions of women dealing with this stage of life. In spite of all the evidence to the contrary—that no woman should "just deal with it" when it comes to menopause— many doctors are still resistant to change when it comes to treating their patients for this stage in their lives.

But the evidence is overwhelming. Today, there are ways for doctors and health-care providers to use HRT to not only safely manage menopause but also reduce numerous health risks associated with aging.

Medical Research

The pages ahead present scientific, thought-changing, cutting-edge information in a way that should help you gain greater understanding of HRT and the health-care landscape today. I'm going to explain the evolution of HRT from decades ago, when we had limited choices, to today, where there are many choices and options.

I'll also talk about some things that we in medicine quite frankly didn't get right. Unfortunately, that happens in medicine as new studies overturn old practices.

Before you delve in, let me first explain a little more about how research works—and how it doesn't.

For starters, it can be difficult to understand what's relevant and what's not. Every day, people are bombarded with information in the media: television, radio, newspaper, online, and even word of mouth. You hear it all the time: "They say you shouldn't eat this." "Everyone says that this helps you lose weight." "Now they're saying that doesn't even work."

But what are the true sources behind all that information (or misinformation)? In some cases, the information may be totally made up or just somebody's best guess. But in many cases, there is science behind the rumors, facts, and innuendos.

It's important to understand that sometimes the discoveries from a scientific study aren't even relevant to your situation. Some studies on animals don't really transfer to humans, other studies only reveal small discoveries that are part of a bigger picture, and some studies jump to the wrong conclusion. Similarly, many of the "weight-loss miracles," "miracle foods," or "miracle cures" are not miracles at all, but sometimes there may be some degree of truth to the hype. Unfortunately, sometimes the wrong information or finding is picked up, disseminated, and widely accepted. Sometimes it's just a matter of how much the information is hyped, how it is spread, or how interesting, exciting, or even bizarre it is.

As discussed earlier, evidence-based medicine is the use of current and contemporaneous information to aid in the practice of medicine. In the introduction, I mentioned how, in my former career of hospital-based medicine, I trained residents how to read medical journals; critically review the information; and then decide whether the information was pertinent and should be practiced, was just steps toward learning how diseases work, or was about the next potential treatment for various conditions.

Today, as part of the evidence-based medicine we practice, there is a plethora of medical journals at our disposal. Decades ago, textbooks were the gold standard for learning and practicing medicine. Then came the proliferation of scientific research and medical journals that are continually updated, making them far more relevant than ten-year-old textbooks. Those medical journals serve as the basis for today's evidence-based medicine.

It's also important to understand the phases that medical research goes through. First, there's a thought, idea, or theory based on some degree of physical or logical evidence. Then a pilot study, involving only a few participants and limited data points, is performed. Once some degree of evidence is identified, these pilot studies tend to expand: more data is collected, more parameters are identified, and more controls are put in place.

Though I won't be diving deeply into the rules of experimentation, you need to understand that doctors may use various therapies and then report their findings, or they may do a clinical experiment that makes a discovery that changes the practice of medicine. Such studies may be conducted first on animals—depending on the potential impact of the treatment, the difficulty of the study, and other factors—or if sufficient evidence exists regarding safety and probability of expected outcomes, the study may be conducted on human beings. Suffice it to say, much novel research is initially performed on animals, and there is usually evidence of benefit over risk by the time things get to human trials.

Types of Studies

There are several types of studies commonly conducted. Understanding each of them can help you decide how much weight should be put on an individual study when forming a conclusion.

Observational studies are conducted to observe a subject's response to a situation, medication, intervention, or other external pressure. These studies often involve a *control*, which is typically either a placebo or a group of matched subjects to which no external pressure is applied. A control helps the researcher determine whether the extra pressure was the likely cause of the outcome.

For instance, a study observing the natural decline in hormones over time wouldn't require controls, because it would just be an observation of increased rates of obesity, diabetes, heart attacks, cancer, or other maladies. Such a study would not establish causation.

However, if we wanted to know whether the decline in hormones *caused* such maladies, then a study might be conducted to look at relative hormone levels or ages at which the decline of hormones occur, along with how those changes affect the aforementioned diseases.

For example, if we discovered that premature ovary failure and the resulting decrease in hormone levels increased incidences of certain diseases, we could guess that it was the lack of hormones that caused the disease. But it's also possible that the condition that led to premature ovary failure also caused the disease (rather than the ovary failure itself being the cause of the disease), so we'd need to conduct a more extensive study to establish the cause.

Although observational studies do not always answer the question "why," they can point out anomalous patterns and can help generate questions to answer.

Randomized control studies involve two groups of subjects with more or less the same characteristics in terms of sex, age, race, weight, etc. In these studies, one group receives one intervention while the other group receives no intervention, a placebo, or a known, baseline treatment. Subjects in these studies are randomly assigned to either the intervention or the placebo group.

An example of a randomized control study might include a group of nonsmoking female college athletes of approximately the same weight and level of activity and with no major medical conditions. The subjects might draw straws to help the researcher determine who gets the supplement that might help them improve their performance and who gets a placebo. The subjects wouldn't see the straws they drew, and in a double-blind study, neither would the researcher. Randomized studies are conducted exhaustively before medications are approved for use, and extensive safety evaluations must be met before they are performed. Yet it is often the preliminary outcomes of these studies that lead to a tremendous amount of hype.

Case-control studies look at some experience and outcome compared to nonexperience and outcome. For case-control studies, researchers look at outcomes first before reviewing the records of the interviews with the patient to see what experiences they had. For example, researchers may look at people with skin cancer and then interview them on their lifetime sun exposure, vitamin D intake, eating habits, smoking history, weight, and other variables. They look at variables that occurred in the life of those with the disease and compare it to those without the disease. This helps predict what experiences increase or decrease the likelihood of different diseases or outcomes.

Review studies: meta-analysis and systematic. A review summarizes literature, studies, and papers produced by others who are more or less trying to make certain assumptions by the aggregate of the knowledge and information. There are two kinds of review studies: *meta-analysis* and *systematic*.

A meta-analysis looks at multiple research studies and combines the findings from those studies to answer a question or an assumption. A meta-analysis might tackle a simple question such as, "Does sunblock prevent skin cancer?" While some studies may show that sunblock doesn't prevent cancer, other studies will show that sunblock has a huge impact. A meta-analysis compares multiple pieces of the research and tries to put them together in a meaningful fashion. For example, it may look at how much sunblock was applied, the sunblock's SPF, its ingredients, subjects' skin color, and so on.

A systematic review also compares multiple scientific papers but on a much broader level than a meta-analysis, often for the sake of general education. For instance, a systematic review on "prevention of skin cancer" may look at different kinds of sunblock, levels of sun exposure, amounts of protective clothing, vitamin levels, skin types, and other factors that may have a bearing on skin cancer and prevention.

Other studies. There are a number of other types of studies that I won't discuss in this book because they do not create proof and are only conducted out of scientific interest. These include case reports, ideas and opinions, and test-tube or bench research.

The pages that follow contain a review of published literature pertinent to the subject. The research presented here has been published in peer-reviewed journals, which are considered the gold standard for publishing medical research: the research has been reviewed by the authors' peers to reveal any bias, inaccurate conclusions, contradictory information, or other inconsistencies.

A list of all papers referenced can be found in the resources section and are available—wholly or in part—through the US National Library of Medicine, part of the National Institutes of Health (NIH).

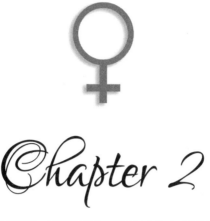

Chapter 2

THE HRT/BREAST CANCER MYTH

The principal reason I wrote this book is because the breast cancer connection to menopause and hormones has been a major source of confusion. There is so much misinformation regarding hormones and breast cancer that it has influenced countless women and their health-care providers to forgo HRT.

Based on what we know now, that decision has been to the detriment of the health of many women. In reality, natural hormone replacement, when done ideally, reduces the risk of breast cancer by up to 75 percent over doing nothing at all for menopause.

The Power of Fear

Breast cancer takes a huge physical and emotional toll when it occurs, not only from the effects disease itself but also from the fear of the disease. The fear of breast cancer has actually *increased* the rate of breast cancer. Let me be clear on this point: we have known for at least two decades how to reduce a woman's chance of breast cancer when in menopause. We have had evidence that HRT, if administered correctly, actually reduces the incidence of breast cancer.

When a couple of large-scale studies—which I'll talk about later in this chapter—conducted some years back showed that a particular form of synthetic hormone replacement increased women's chance of breast cancer, the reaction in the medical community and among the public was so strong that virtually every doctor and patient abandoned or considered abandoning hormone replacement.

At the time, there were other, often ignored, studies showing how to mitigate breast cancer risk with hormone replacement, and there were flaws in one of the impactful studies that linked HRT with increased breast cancer in the first place. Again, a flawed study of synthetic HRT that showed a slight increase in the risk of breast cancer had far greater impact than other studies, which showed decreases in breast cancer when natural hormone replacement was used. That's how the fear of breast cancer has increased its incidence; beneficial, natural HRT was abandoned out of a misguided fear, leaving women to suffer.

Going a step further, we have had evidence for several years now that proper hormone replacement not only can protect women from breast cancer but *can actually reduce the rate of breast cancer by more than 50 to 75 percent.* Yet the medical community is still slow to adapt.

Breast Cancer—the Facts

According to the American Cancer Society, breast cancer is the second-most common form of cancer in women. Skin cancer is the most common form of cancer in women, but it is less serious in most cases.

Invasive breast cancer occurs in about one out of eight women, most often during menopause. The occurrence is slightly higher with noninvasive (in situ) breast cancer, which grows in the milk duct and does not involve other breast tissues. In situ cancers are commonly referred to as "precancer" because they stay in a local area and are not invasive.

Each year, about a quarter of a million women will develop invasive breast cancer, and another sixty thousand will develop in situ (nonnvasive) breast cancer.

Women with a first-degree relative with a history of breast cancer have twice the risk of developing cancer themselves, yet a majority (85 percent) of women with newly diagnosed breast cancer have no immediate family members with the disease.

Two genes—BRCA1 and BRCA2—double a woman's risk of breast cancer, yet they only account for 5 to 10 percent of all newly diagnosed breast cancer.

By far the biggest risk factors for developing breast cancer are being female (a hundred times more likely than men) and age. Therefore, women of menopausal age have two major strikes against them.

While these facts can be somewhat alarming, look at the bigger picture: the majority of women will never get breast cancer. Still, with the risk factors being so prevalent, it's certainly a good idea to look at preventive measures to reduce any undue risk.

While no preventive measures can guarantee you will not get breast cancer, the National Cancer Institute and others publish evidence that following healthy living guidelines reduce the risk. These guidelines include the following:

- having children and breastfeeding before age thirty

- moderate to vigorous exercise four to seven hours each week
- getting enough vitamin D
- reducing artificial light at night

There is also considerable evidence that eating healthily can reduce your breast cancer risk. Increasing your intake of fruit and vegetables can lower your risk, as can limiting your intake of processed meats (cold cuts, ham, jerky, bacon), red meat, and—surprisingly—grilled meats. Because there are also links between cancer and compounds such as pesticides, preservatives, and mercury, eating organic foods will likely reduce your risk, even though *organic* is not a clearly defined term. Certain organic fruits and vegetables are better choices because they are grown without conventional pesticides or fertilizers, but their role in breast cancer prevention is not clear. With meats, there is clear evidence that "grass-fed" or "pasture-raised" is better for you than "grain-fed." And with fish, wild-caught, nonpredatory fish are healthier than farmed fish or fish that eat other fish.

Where It Went Wrong

The idea for HRT was a good one from the start. But along the way, things went very wrong.

Prior to 2002, it was fairly common for all women to be offered hormone replacements after menopause. Earlier studies clearly showed there were numerous health benefits to HRT. Many of these studies used a combination of some type of estrogen (commonly horse estrogen) and either natural progesterone or synthetic progestin, which was a drug designed to protect the uterus from stimulation by estrogen.

A large trial in the 1990s called the PEPI (Postmenopausal Estrogen/Progestin Interventions) was designed largely to determine the effects of HRT on the heart and lipids, which are the standard units currently used to measure risk (HDL and LDL cholesterols, C-reactive protein made in the liver, and others). The conclusion was that HRT not only helped the symptoms of menopause but was also beneficial for the cardiovascular system.

Then in mid-2002, the *Journal of the American Medical Association* published the results of one of the WHI clinical trials. The trial involved more than sixteen thousand postmenopausal women taking horse estrogen with or without synthetic progestin for more than eight years. In the trial, one group of women took CEE (horse estrogen) plus medroxyprogesterone acetate (a synthetic progestin) while the other group took a placebo. The study found that "all-cause mortality" was the same between the treated groups and the controls, meaning that death rates were the same in both groups. There was a slightly greater risk (eight in ten thousand) of heart disease, stroke, blood clots, and breast cancer, and slightly lessened risk (six to seven fewer cases per ten thousand) of colorectal cancer and hip fractures.

• •

The HRT Evolution

1940s HRT: Horse estrogen alone.

1970s HRT: Horse estrogen plus progesterone—worked well and reduced uterine cancer.

1980s HRT: Horse estrogen plus synthetic progestin. It became standard to prescribe HRT for most women in menopause, particularly for cardiac prevention.

1990s HRT: Horse estrogen is the number-one drug prescribed in the US for next two decades.

2002s HRT: Increased risk of breast cancer in women taking horse estrogen with synthetic progestin. HRT prescriptions drop precipitously.

2010s HRT: Greater than 50 percent reduction in risk of breast cancer and reduction of all menopause symptoms in women taking testosterone. Very little need for estrogen.

• •

What's important about the landmark WHI trials is that they led to a substantial change in how symptoms of menopause were managed. Even though the WHI trials did not replicate the common practice of medicine at the time, they had an enormous negative impact. I'll talk about this more later, but in summary, the WHI trials prescribed synthetic hormones to women who had already been in menopause for some time instead at the onset of menopause, which is the usual practice. This timing issue had a major impact on the outcomes of the therapy.

Two years after the results of the trial were released, the results of another of the WHI's trials were published. This trial looked at women who had undergone a hysterectomy and included only horse estrogen—no progestin, because progestin is designed to protect the uterus from continuous exposure to estrogen (which would lead to bleeding and possibly uterine cancer). The results of this trial showed a slightly increased risk of stroke, fewer hip fractures, and no effect on the rest of the cardiovascular system. It also revealed a *trend toward risk reduction in breast cancer,* demonstrating that women on estrogen alone, even horse-based estrogen, saw no increases in breast cancer. The problems that arose in the other study, it appears, were largely related to the synthetic progestin, an artificial copy of the hormone progesterone.

Occurring around the same time as the US-based WHI trials was a study in the United Kingdom known as the "Million Women Study." The results of this study were reported in *The Lancet*, a major UK medical publication. The massive report reviewed the history of randomly recruited women—yes, approximately a million women participated—aged fifty to sixty-four, paying special attention to their HRT use and incidence of breast cancer. This observational study did not randomize the medications used, and there was no placebo control.

The findings of The Million Women Study were similar to the WHI trials: Women who took an estrogen plus a synthetic progestin had a statistically significant higher rate of breast cancer than women taking estrogen alone. However, the study also found a slightly increased risk of developing breast cancer (about 0.5 to 1 percent) when taking any form of estrogen, with or without synthetic progestin.

The Million Women Study has been criticized because the increased observed risk of breast cancer was so small that it may have been random chance, but nonetheless, it was very concerning. Another study done on women from Finland looked at the rates of breast cancer for women on estrogen only and found that for women taking HRT for greater than five years, there was a 0.0025 percent increase in the rate of breast cancer as well. This small increase in risk may not seem substantial until we consider the millions of women taking these prescriptions annually. And the rates of relative risk may be different between the studies because of unknown geographic and contributing factors, as well as the study designs—not all were following women using the exact same synthetic hormones.

While the absolute increased risk is minuscule, the obvious public-health issues are enormous when you consider the billions of women who will need to decide on management options when they enter menopause.

I will now discuss where other trials got it wrong and the difference between these studies and the myriad of favorable options that women have for menopause treatment.

Mistake #1: Using a nonhuman, synthetic progestin instead of natural progesterone

Again, synthetic progestin appeared to be the likely causative factor for the slight increase in the rate of breast cancer when used with estrogen. Natural progesterone, which is a hormone and not a drug, does not have this undesirable risk.

Another variable entered the discussion of HRT safety when in 2013, a large study involving women in France was published. In France, it is common to use micronized progesterone instead of a synthetic progestin. Micronized progesterone is a plant-based (known as a *bioidentical*) version of naturally occurring progesterone. The French study observed that there was no increased incidence of breast cancer when natural progesterone was used.

So the pattern emerged that estrogen alone may or may not increase the incidence of breast cancer but that very likely, synthetic progestin does increase that risk.

Another French study from 1999 found that subjects taking both natural estrogen and progesterone had fewer incidences of breast cancer, while those taking estrogen and synthetic progestin had more incidences of breast cancer. The implication may be that progestin can stimulate breast cancer and progesterone can block it. This finding may be further supported by a 2008 French study that found taking estrogen alone or with a synthetic progestin increased breast cancer rates, while taking estrogen with natural progesterone did not.

Complicating the issue further was a 1997 study in Sweden that found a more favorable prognoses for women who were on HRT and were diagnosed with breast cancer than women not on HRT in whom breast cancer was discovered. These findings, however, could be biased because the women on HRT were seeing a physician and were therefore more likely to have a screening that led to earlier detection and, thus, better outcomes.

In summary, synthetic progestin (and perhaps estrogen, to a lesser degree) likely increases a woman's chance of getting breast cancer. Natural progesterone, however, decreases that risk.

Mistake #2: Choosing the wrong hormone to replace

Maybe we just picked the wrong primary hormone (estrogen) to start with for the treatment of menopause.

The assumption for decades was that symptoms of menopause were caused by the absence of estrogen. In fact, early treatments of menopause used estrogen only, until it was discovered that estrogen alone could increase risk of uterine cancer. Progesterone and synthetic progestin were added to reduce that risk.

The goal of all the treatments was to reduce or eliminate the symptoms of menopause, which include but are not limited to the following:

- hot flashes
- sweating
- sleep problems
- moodiness
- irritability/anxiety
- fatigue

- joint and muscle pain
- bladder symptoms
- decreased sexual desire, activity, and satisfaction
- loss of thickness and fullness of scalp hair
- decreased bone density
- memory loss
- vaginal dryness

Again, these symptoms can be improved with HRT but potentially at the cost of increased incidence of breast cancer—particularly when using synthetic drugs.

What all of the studies missed was another key hormone in a woman's body.

Testosterone: Strong Enough for a Man, Also Made for a Woman

Testosterone is another hormone that is present in healthy young women and at a *concentration that is five to twenty times greater than estrogen*. Factoring in other androgens, which are a group of testosterone-like hormones, the ratio is even greater.

Initially, testosterone therapy was used for libido, mood, well-being, and sexual satisfaction. With the concerns over estrogen and synthetic progestin increasing breast cancer risk, there were initial concerns that testosterone replacement could do the same thing.

Without testosterone, there is no estrogen. A woman's body requires androgens (which I'll refer to as *testosterone* for simplicity's sake) to make estrogen.

Some studies looking at estrogen-to-testosterone ratios have led scientists to believe that testosterone replacement for women could have negative consequences. But these were observational studies that ultimately seemed to suggest that other illnesses and conditions—obesity, metabolic syndrome, diabetes, polycystic ovarian syndrome, heart disease, and so on—caused extremely unnatural ratios of estrogen to testosterone. The high-baseline measurement of testosterone in women with these and other conditions led to a false assumption about testosterone's negative impact. So the relationship between testosterone levels and breast cancer has been all over the map.

Adding to the confusion is the problematic nature of blood testing of hormones, where numerous factors such as variable molecules, time of day, hormonal interplay, and external stressors play a role in results. Consequently, some practitioners look at salivary levels of hormones, which are in a steadier state because they are not influenced by the aforementioned factors. Salivary testing is useful for baseline measurements but is limited in that the saliva is altered by the replacement therapy itself.

One study that used salivary samples to determine baseline hormone levels produced some interesting results. The study looked at the sexual hormones of women with breast cancer and used women who did not have cancer as a control. The study's participants were matched for age, family history of breast cancer, menopause status, use of HRT, age at menarche, and age at first birth. If they had been on HRT, they had to be off the therapy for two months prior to testing to avoid any interference.

The hormone levels of 357 women with breast cancer and a nearly equal number of women without breast cancer were tested. Testing was performed first thing in the morning so that daytime swings would not influence the results. The study found that women with breast cancer had lower testosterone as well as lower DHEA-S levels. Like testosterone, DHEA-S is a hormone that suppresses breast cancer cell proliferation. The subjects with breast cancer were also found to have lower estriol, which is considered a protective estrogen and is commonly used as a treatment for vaginal dryness or dry skin. Estriol is elevated in pregnancy and is a major hormone at that time, not be confused with the major estrogen, estradiol, spelled with a "d".

In the study of baseline hormone levels, women with breast cancer also had higher levels of the major estrogen estradiol and of estrone, of which some subtypes have been strongly associated with breast cancer. Interestingly, progesterone levels were pretty much the same between the groups, as were cortisol levels. Cancer patients with higher-than-average testosterone also tended to have higher-than-average estradiol. In these cases where the testosterone was increased, the increase in estrogen was triple the rate of increase of testosterone, indicating that hormone levels alone don't link to the development of breast cancer—the ratio also factors in.

Another interesting aspect of the study was that it looked at both cancer and "carcinoma in situ," or precancer. Again, the study suggested that estrogen-to-testosterone ratio predicted the possible development of cancer but was less able to predict proliferation of cancers.

This and other studies led to the concept that that the addition of testosterone to HRT may reduce or negate HRT as a risk factor for breast cancer. As a result, an entirely new approach to managing menopause emerged; instead of looking solely at estrogen as a treatment for women in menopause, testosterone replacement began to also be considered.

Testosterone: Plenty to Go Around

While hormone ratios are different between the sexes, the fact remains that healthy young women have up to twenty times more testosterone than estrogen, and men have twenty times more testosterone than women.

Testosterone is produced in a woman's ovary, just like estrogen, but there's a lot more of it. A look at a blood-work report may not reveal a ratio—10:1 or 20:1—but it will reveal two very different units of measure.

Hormone units on lab reports are typically measured as ng/dl(nanograms per deciliter) and pg/ml (picograms per milliliter). Ten pg/ml equals one ng/dl.

Consider this example of an actual lab test on a fifty-two-year-old female.
Testosterone: 62 ng/dl
Estradiol: 30 pg/ml

To make the units the same
Testosterone 620 pg/ml and estradiol 30 pg/ml
or
Testosterone 62 ng/dl and estradiol 0.3 ng/dl
In both cases, it is 20:1.

Blocking Estrogen's Breast Stimulatory Effects

Estrogen stimulates the breast tissue. This may be why estrogen combined with synthetic progestin leads to slightly more breast cancer. But testosterone does the opposite. It reduces estrogen receptors and blocks estrogen's stimulatory effect on the breast and does so even better than anticancer drugs.

Over the past two decades, animal and human studies have looked at the effect of testosterone on breast tissue and breast cancer. For the most part, these studies have shown that while estrogen typically stimulates breast cancer cell growth, testosterone inhibits cancer growth and can actually cause the cancer cells to die. Stimulation of breast tissue is the precursor to the development of breast cancer. These studies found numerous contributing factors, such as relative concentrations of androgens, type of cancer, cancer receptors, and others. But they built a scientific basis for the investigation of testosterone's role in breast cancer. They also left unanswered questions such as this prominent one: Given that testosterone turns into estrogen, then even if it suppresses breast cancer, can it also stimulate cancer when it is converted to estrogen?

Animal Studies Show Testosterone Blocks Stimulation

A 2000 study of female monkeys with removed ovaries was divided into five groups: placebo, estradiol (the dominant estrogen in females), estradiol plus progestin, estradiol plus testosterone, and estradiol plus tamoxifen. Tamoxifen is a synthetic estrogen receptor modulator used to treat or prevent breast cancer in women at risk. Receptors are molecules in or on the surface of cells that take cues from other substances in the bloodstream. When a substance in the bloodstream binds to a cell receptor, it signals the cell to perform an activity, typically to grow or send out a signal to activate some other function in the body.

Breast tissue biopsies of those receiving treatment were compared to baseline (before medications) samples and those from the placebo group.

The estrogen-only group experienced a 600 percent increase in breast cell proliferation, while estrogen receptors increased by 50 percent. In other words, the estrogen stimulated breast tissue growth and also upped the ability of the breast cells to "see" the hormone.

In the estrogen-plus-progestin group, the addition of progestin did not stop the breast cell proliferation nor did it prevent the growth of new receptors.

The estrogen-plus-tamoxifen group saw a 300 percent increase in breast cell proliferation—less than the estrogen alone—and a decrease in the estrogen receptors.

The estrogen-plus-testosterone group experienced both a 40 percent decrease in breast cell proliferation and no increase in estrogen receptors. So, unlike tamoxifen, the testosterone worked at both levels.

This study showed that testosterone is far superior at preventing breast tissue growth than current breast cancer drugs. Testosterone basically turned off stimulation of breast tissue.

In 2002, another study was performed on female monkeys to answer the question of whether breast cell proliferation from estrogen and progestin (and thereby, development of breast cancer) could be stopped by the addition of testosterone. The monkeys had no ovaries and were divided into four groups: placebo; estrogen; estrogen plus synthetic progestin; and estrogen, synthetic progestin, and testosterone.

Breast tissue biopsies in both the estrogen and the estrogen-plus-progestin groups showed a 350 percent increase of breast tissue proliferation over the baseline biopsy. In the control (placebo) and estrogen, progestin, and testosterone groups, there was no significant change in breast cell proliferation.

This study shows that estrogen stimulates the breast tissue, and testosterone completely blocks that stimulation.

Human Studies Show Testosterone Blocks Breast Cell Proliferation from Estrogen

If testosterone can reduce breast cell stimulation and cancer in animals, what about humans?

In 2006, a Swedish study looked at whether adding testosterone to the usual estrogen and synthetic progestin preparations stimulated breast tissue differently compared to estrogen and progesterone alone.

In this study, menopausal-symptomatic and laboratory-proven-menopausal women were given estradiol plus a progestin. The women were divided into two groups: half wore a placebo patch, and the other half wore a patch containing testosterone. Breast biopsies performed after six months found a five-fold increase in breast cell proliferation in the women on estrogen and synthetic progestin alone and no increase in the women treated with testosterone in addition to estrogen and synthetic progestin.

This was the first human study showing that testosterone specifically blocked breast tissue proliferation (growth and activity), which is when breast cancer tends to develop.

The Breast Cancer Blocker?

Testosterone, when added to HRT or used alone, substantially blocks the development of breast cancer.

The studies I've discussed here have shown how testosterone is very effective in blocking the stimulatory effect of estrogen on the breast tissue. Now let's look at studies that show testosterone to be very effective at blocking the development of breast cancer itself.

First, let me explain a term to help you better understand these studies. *Person-years* is a comparative statistics term that is essentially the total amount of time that the subjects in a study have been exposed to specified conditions. For instance, a hundred smokers in a two-year study equals two hundred person-years. This unit of measure allows for comparison of study results. For instance, if one study showed that the risk of cancer was thirty in three thousand person-years (expressed as 30/3,000), while another study using a miracle drug showed that the risk of cancer was ten in three thousand person-years (10/3,000), then the knowns of the study would be that the number of people and time were similar. But questions might still be raised: What were the ages of the subjects in the two groups? What was the exposure rate of the two groups?

Also, it needs to be clear that when it comes to testosterone replacement therapy, more research needs to be conducted, particularly so that the results can be dissected and real comparisons can be made.

For now, let's look at the latest research of testosterone and breast cancer in groups of women of the same age. These studies provide evidence that testosterone is critical in menopause not only to improve quality of life but also to provide remarkable protection against breast cancer.

In the WHI trial and some of the other studies I've discussed, the rate of breast cancer was 380 to 520 cases per 100,000 person-years.

An Australian study published two years after the WHI trials was conducted over a span of eight years and showed a breast cancer rate of 293 per 100,000 person-years. This study looked at the rate of breast cancer in women taking estrogen (either horse estrogen or estradiol) plus a progestin along with a testosterone pellet. A hormone pellet is a rice-sized dose, placed under the skin, which dissolves over three to five months' time. The advantage of the pellet is that the delivery is consistent, and you don't have to remember to use a patch or cream. I'll talk more about the pellet and other hormone-delivery systems later in the book.

The results of this study found a 380/100,000 person-years rate of breast cancer for women on estrogen plus progestin and a 293/100,000 person-years rate of breast cancer in women on a combination of estrogen, progestin, and testosterone. Adding testosterone caused a 24 percent decline in expected rates of breast cancer.

This and other studies raise the question of whether the addition of testosterone alone is enough to reduce the risk of breast cancer. To answer that question, researchers looked at other factors that occur when HRT is administered. For instance, when conventional hormones such as estrogen are used, there is a subsequent natural feedback mechanism that leads to the production of fewer androgens (such as testosterone) and increased production of sex hormone binding globulin (SHBG). SHBG is produced in response to estrogen, and it in turn reduces free-circulating testosterone. This is particularly true when the estrogen is taken in pill form, as opposed to a patch, where the first-pass effect occurs; the *first-pass effect* refers to the reduced effectiveness of a medication due to its being highly metabolized before it is sufficiently circulated through the body.

SHBG has a stronger affinity for testosterone and other androgens than for estrogen. When SHBG sponges up hormones, the effect is less free-circulating testosterone, which is a breast cancer protector.

So not only do certain estrogen replacements (as well as synthetic progestin replacement) slightly increase your risk of breast cancer, they also suppress your own testosterone, which is a breast cancer blocker.

The Dayton Study

The Dayton study showed that using testosterone (as a tiny, implanted pellet) for women in menopause ultimately led to over 70 percent reduction in the rates of breast cancer.

The Dayton study was a landmark study initiated in Dayton, Ohio, in 2008 to determine if testosterone inserted as a pellet would, by itself, reduce incidence of breast cancer below predicted levels. There was already sufficient evidence that testosterone would reduce breast cancer if added to conventional hormone replacement, but this study ultimately led to the transition of my practice in treating menopause. Today, we treat all women presenting with menopause systems with testosterone because the evidence is now overwhelming.

Prior to the Dayton study, there was evidence suggesting that testosterone plus an estrogen blocker relieved symptoms of menopause and that women being treated for breast cancer with estrogen blockers had better symptom relief when testosterone treatment was added.

While the study was originally planned to last ten years, its preliminary data was presented after five years, in 2013. Participants in the study presented a variety of hormone deficiency symptoms including hot flashes and sweating, sleep disturbances and fatigue, anxiety and irritability, heart discomfort and depression, memory loss and migraines, premenstrual syndrome, sexual problems (including vaginal dryness), urinary symptoms (including incontinence), bone loss, and musculoskeletal pain.

The control group was composed of women who chose not to participate in testosterone therapy. Two other groups were treated for their symptoms with testosterone. One group received testosterone pellets, and the other group received testosterone pellets with anastrozole, a drug that blocks the conversion of testosterone into estrogen.

Table 1

Indications for aromatase inhibitor therapy in female patients

History of breast cancer
_____

Increased risk for breast cancer

    Atypical ductal hyperplasia

    Strong family history

    Lobular carcinoma in situ

Severe fibrocystic breast tissue, breast pain

Endometriosis, uterine fibroids, dysfunctional uterine bleeding

Weight gain, increased abdominal obesity/fat

Insulin resistance, metabolic syndrome with elevated estradiol

Menstrual or migraine headaches

PMS, anxiety, irritability, aggression, fluid retention, bloating

Adapted from the 9th European Congress on Menopause and Andropause [10].

The five-year data showed improvements across all aspects of the menopause rating scale. The data also showed that the women on testosterone or testosterone plus estrogen blocker had a risk of breast cancer of 142/100,000 person-years, compared to the control group's breast cancer rate of 390/100,000 person-years. But the real take-home points are that there was a greater than 50 percent reduction in the rate of breast cancer with testosterone replacement without estrogen and that testosterone alone reduces all symptoms of menopause.

Menopause Rating Scale (MRS)

Which of the following symptoms apply to you at this time? Please, mark the appropriate box for each symptom. For symptoms that do not apply, please mark 'none'.

Symptoms:

		none	mild	moderate	severe	very severe
	Score =	0	1	2	3	4
1.	Hot flushes, sweating (episodes of sweating)	☐	☐	☐	☐	☐
2.	Heart discomfort (unusual awareness of heart beat, heart skipping, heart racing, tightness)	☐	☐	☐	☐	☐
3.	Sleep problems (difficulty in falling asleep, difficulty in sleeping through, waking up early)	☐	☐	☐	☐	☐
4.	Depressive mood (feeling down, sad, on the verge of tears, lack of drive, mood swings)	☐	☐	☐	☐	☐
5.	Irritability (feeling nervous, inner tension, feeling aggressive)	☐	☐	☐	☐	☐
6.	Anxiety (inner restlessness, feeling panicky)	☐	☐	☐	☐	☐
7.	Physical and mental exhaustion (general decrease in performance, impaired memory, decrease in concentration, forgetfulness)	☐	☐	☐	☐	☐
8.	Sexual problems (change in sexual desire, in sexual activity and satisfaction)	☐	☐	☐	☐	☐
9.	Bladder problems (difficulty in urinating, increased need to urinate, bladder incontinence)	☐	☐	☐	☐	☐
10.	Dryness of vagina (sensation of dryness or burning in the vagina, difficulty with sexual intercourse)	☐	☐	☐	☐	☐
11.	Joint and muscular discomfort (pain in the joints, rheumatoid complaints)	☐	☐	☐	☐	☐

The five-year study showed a 50 percent reduction in breast cancer, improvements in all symptoms of menopause, and no adverse drug effects using testosterone pellets without estrogen.

• •

Susan: Taking Better Care of Self

In her midfifties, Susan started "feeling her age." "I was tired a lot, and I was feeling old," she said. "I was putting on weight, and I had no initiative to do anything."

Since she had been treated at Allure for varicose veins a few years prior, she reached out to see if Allure offered HRT and was delighted to find out it did. "I liked Dr. Mok and the people at Allure; I really liked how they worked and how they treated patients, so they were my first choice," she said. "They ask you a lot of questions, and they want to know the reason that you're there and the problems you're having that you want resolved. They're genuinely concerned and want you to get results."

She made an appointment to discuss HRT, and after blood work confirmed what hormone levels were low, she was put on a treatment of testosterone cream and capsules. When Allure started offering pellets, she opted for the implants instead. "The pellets are much more convenient; I don't have to think about them," she said.

Within a month of taking the first treatment, she wanted to take better care of herself. Inspired to lose weight, she got on a weight-loss program and started exercising. The result? A seventy-pound weight loss. "And my husband says I'm not crabby anymore," she said.

• •

Use of Testosterone beyond Five Years

The Dayton study also followed women beyond the initial five years, during which time most of the participants received testosterone as the sole hormone for menopause relief. For women with risk factors such as a family history of breast pain or a personal history of breast pain, breast symptoms, uterine bleeding, obesity, or elevated estradiol levels, an estrogen blocker was added. The result was that 95 percent of women had relief of all symptoms of menopause with testosterone alone. Only 5 percent of women failed to have adequate menopause symptom relief with just testosterone, so that 5 percent had estrogen added.

A couple of years later, the breast cancer rate dropped further, to 76/100,000 person-years. This group was called the *adherent group*, which means that they stayed with the program for the duration. In this group, with testosterone alone, there was a continued decline of around 75 percent of breast cancer risk.

So testosterone relieves the symptoms of menopause, has no major adverse effects, and reduces your risk of developing breast cancer. Plus, the longer you take testosterone, the more breast cancer protection you have.

Breast Cancer Prevention

Today, if you are concerned about developing breast cancer because of genetic risk factors, you may be offered a drug such as tamoxifen, or you may opt for surgical removal of the breasts in cases of very high risk.

Long-term studies show that tamoxifen is 29 percent effective at reducing rates of breast cancer. However, it comes with a few side effects:

- thirty-five to fifty percent loss of bone mass, which can lead to more life-threatening fractures
- increase in the incidence of endometrial cancer
- vaginal dryness, low libido, hot flashes, mood swings, nausea

In other words, though tamoxifen can reduce the risk of breast cancer in high-risk women by 29 percent, but it also increases the symptoms of menopause. That compares to a 75 percent breast cancer risk reduction with testosterone. Additionally, testosterone has no major adverse effects and improves all symptoms of menopause.

Testosterone Replacement for Breast Cancer Survivors

Because testosterone has proven so beneficial in combating menopause symptoms and breast cancer, other studies have looked at testosterone to treat symptoms of menopause in breast cancer survivors.

In one study, seventy-two women who had survived breast cancer and had menopause symptoms were given pellets of testosterone along with an estrogen blocker. An aromatase inhibitor was included in the testosterone pellet to prevent the testosterone from converting into estrogen. The women in the study had survived various stages of cancer, from 0 to 4, with stage 0 being the least severe cancer and stage 4 being advanced and metastatic—the most serious type.

The women were evaluated for symptoms of menopause such as anxiety and depression, mental and physical exhaustion, hot flashes, sleep problems, decreased sexual satisfaction, vaginal dryness, and urinary issues, and they rated their menopause severity on a scale of 1 (mild) to 10 (severe).

The results of the study showed that the women were able to achieve therapeutic testosterone levels with no rise in estrogen levels. So instead of being given an estrogen blocker that would have worsened their quality of life, the treatment with testosterone actually improved their menopausal symptoms. And there was no recurrence of cancer after nine years.

Breast Cancer Severity

If a woman has breast cancer, her risk of living five years without recurrence is based on the stage of the cancer. The stage is basically the severity when detected on testing.

- **Stage 0:** In situ; a precancer in the milk duct or a tumor < 5 mm (pea size) when detected.
- **Stage 1:** Tumor < 2 cm (postage-stamp size); no cancer in the lymph nodes.
- **Stages 2 and 3:** Lymph nodes are involved. This is critical because diseased lymph nodes indicate the cancer is trying to spread in the body.
- **Stage 4:** Metastasis. The cancer has spread to other organs. This is by far the most serious.

Conventional Treatment

Here are the relative rates of cancer recurrence with conventional cancer treatment intervention. Rates represent a five-year period. Ten-year statistics are a little worse for stages 0–3 and much worse for stage 4.

- **Stage 0:** 98 percent cancer free
- **Stage 1:** 85 percent cancer free
- **Stages 2 and 3:** 55 percent cancer free

- **Stage 4:** 10 percent cancer free (2 percent cancer free at ten years)

Testosterone for Existing Breast Cancer

The use of testosterone for breast cancer suppression is a relatively new discovery.

In breast cancer (or any cancer), the cells mutate and can grow excessively. With breast cancer, there is an overabundance of aromatase, the component that converts circulating hormones into estrogen, which stimulates the cancer to grow. As the tumor makes more estrogen, it tends to grow faster; the nature of aggressive tumors is the ability to help themselves grow.

• •

100 Percent Cancer Free

In the testosterone-plus-estrogen-blocker study, women with breast cancer stages 0–4 had no recurrence at 9.4 years.

• •

Case Report: Testosterone Reverses Existing Breast Cancer

In 2013, a ninety-year-old, healthy woman was the first reported case of breast cancer actually being reversed with testosterone along with an estrogen blocker.

The woman received the treatment after having been found to have a sizable breast cancer mass. It was recommended that she undergo surgery followed by treatment with tamoxifen, which was a standard therapy for her situation. She declined the surgery, which is not unusual for a woman her age, but she was open to the idea of taking anticancer medication. No changes occurred with the tumor after four months, so she was offered testosterone therapy.

She had been on chemotherapy but discontinued it and was given testosterone and estrogen-blocking implants in pellet form. However, instead of placing the pellets in the hip or buttocks, as is common, three pellets were placed in a way that surrounded the cancer.

Over two to four weeks, the tumor shrunk, and the pain associated with it relaxed.

At six weeks, the tumor had shrunk 85 percent; at thirteen weeks, it had shrunk 92 percent!

The patient also had better memory, had fewer sleep problems, and just felt better overall. She was also able to cut down on blood-pressure medications. And even more exciting, she was able to put aside her walker and start driving a car again.

• •

The Winning Edge

- Estrogen is linked to breast cancer, which remains a significant public-health concern, affecting one in every eight women in their lifetime. There is evidence that the type of estrogen may have a small impact on the rates of breast cancer.

- Progesterone is likely slightly breast cancer protective. If a woman takes any form of estrogen, from a breast cancer perspective, she is better off taking actual progesterone (the hormone) than a synthetic progestin (a drug).

- Testosterone, which is thought of as a "male hormone," is in fact the dominant sex hormone in young, healthy women; however, it declines with age. Testosterone decreases breast cell proliferation and reduces estrogen receptors in breast tissue in the face of estrogen therapy.

- Nearly every woman will experience symptoms of menopause, but testosterone treats all symptoms of menopause and sex hormone imbalance with no significant adverse side effects. It clearly reduces the chance of developing breast cancer, and it may actually treat or cure breast cancer.

- Selecting estrogen for menopause treatment is where we got it wrong in the past. Estrogen works but comes with health risks when taken alone. The addition of testosterone led to a reduction of breast cancer and improved symptom relief: 95 percent of women get relief of menopause symptoms with testosterone alone. Testosterone reduces the risk of breast cancer dramatically, and the longer it's taken, the more protection from breast cancer you have.

- Testosterone also improves all symptoms of menopause and has other quality-of-life and disease-prevention benefits, as well.

• •

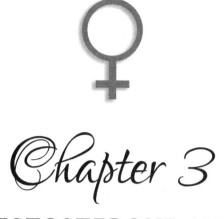

Chapter 3

TESTOSTERONE AND SEXUAL HEALTH

Beyond its crucial role for women in perimenopause and menopause and in preventing and potentially even curing breast cancer, testosterone is also an essential hormone for women's sexual health.

In our practice, we emphasize women's sexual health as well as overall well-being. We were one of the first practices in the nation to offer treatments for orgasm dysfunction with a minor, nonsurgical procedure commonly known as *G-spot amplification*. This treatment involves injecting a filler—the same as used for treating deflation of the aging face—into the area of the G-spot. A majority of women we treat experience deep vaginal orgasms more frequently and with less effort than before the treatment.

We also treat vaginal relaxation syndrome and urinary stress incontinence with modern, novel, nonsurgical, laser-based devices. Vaginal relaxation can occur from childbirth or with natural aging. The laser tightens the tissue. The vast majority of women treated see an immediate improvement in sexual stimulation and sensation and more frequent orgasms—many become multiple orgasmic. Sexual satisfaction is improved in almost all women who undergo this minor, in-office, nonsurgical treatment. Urinary stress incontinence improves in the vast majority of women with only one treatment.

Because of this practice, we are trying to stay tuned in to issues with women's sexuality and are able to frankly and openly discuss this in an unintimidating fashion. It is an inherent part of our practice. Yet outside our walls, we still see an amazing bias by the medical community against women's sexuality.

To demonstrate, let me share with you a little recent history.

In 2004, the Food and Drug Administration (FDA) advisory panel, which oversees the safety and efficacy of drugs prior to their release to the US market, voted unanimously to deny a drug company the right to make a testosterone patch that was shown to benefit women with sexual dysfunction. The reason cited: lack of long-term proof of safety.

At the time, there was plenty of long-term proof, and the bias exhibited by the medical community toward women's sexual health was nothing short of astounding. In this chapter, I'll share with you additional stories of the sheer audacity of doctors and medical groups that have viewed female sexual health as a nonissue that carries no weight or value or who have denied that it even exists!

It's a glaring contradiction, as evidenced by the number of options on the market. Men can currently choose from Viagra, Cialis, and Levitra for erectile dysfunction. In fact, it only took two years for Pfizer to get FDA approval for Viagra after discovering in 1996 it was a potential treatment for erectile dysfunction. That's two years from discovery to release to market. It's unheard of for a drug to be researched, patented, and approved by the FDA in that span of time—it commonly takes five times that long. And long-term safety wasn't even a requirement by the FDA.

Eventually the FDA approved a drug for women to treat sexual health. After much urging by Congress, the FDA eventually approved Addyi®, a drug for female sexual desire, even though it doesn't work well and has potential side effects. This drug is also not nearly as safe or effective as testosterone, which has had a proven track record for decades.

Testosterone for Better Health

Contrary to conventional medical opinion, sexual dysfunction does occur in women. With a loss of sensitivity and satisfaction and a decrease in the ability to experience orgasms, women can find themselves desiring sexual activity less often. That's where testosterone comes in.

Again, testosterone is a crucial hormone for women. It is in a class of hormones called androgens, which both men and women have. Men have about ten times more testosterone than women, and women have five to twenty times more testosterone than they have estrogen. Estrogen is made from testosterone and other androgens in a process called aromatization, where an enzyme alters the testosterone very slightly and turns it into estrogen.

Testosterone is made largely in the ovaries and the adrenal glands, but its production falls with age—a little each year after age twenty. Unlike estrogen, testosterone levels do not fall precipitously during menopause; the decline is gradual, except in the case of a hysterectomy with ovary removal. When the ovaries are removed, the drop in testosterone is sudden, and symptoms of low testosterone appear rapidly. Prior to menopause, women may also experience less sexual desire and fulfillment as a result of what's known as *androgen deficiency*.

In fact, initial studies involving testosterone in women were focused on the relationship of androgen hormones to sexual desire and satisfaction. A quick look at the major medical research databases—PubMed, US National Library of Medicine—reveals more than a thousand studies aimed at evaluating testosterone and sexual function in women.

Among these is a position statement published in 2005 in the medical journal *Menopause: The Journal of the North American Menopause Society*. A position statement is a clear consensus directing doctors and practitioners to the best practice for a given disease. Position statements are designed to eliminate controversy in the medical community, in that they are generally formulated after years of research and proof have been developed and published and there has been a sustained review of best practices and extensive literature review. Position statements carry a lot of weight, and we doctors are supposed to regard them based on the time they are released. A doctor who is aware of a position statement may be able to offer more up-to-date medicine.

The aforementioned position statement referenced sixty-six peer-reviewed medical research papers and concluded that "postmenopausal women with decreased sexual desire associated with personal distress and with no other identifiable cause may be candidates for testosterone therapy."

Interestingly, after the original (now-retired) position statement was released, it was attacked by the medical community for addressing sexual health with medical therapy instead of with traditional, less-effective psychosocial therapy. Other societies went on to criticize this position statement as a "craze in the post-Viagra era."

The criticism was consistent with the medical establishment's view of women's sexuality: "It's all in their head, it's not a condition of declining hormones, the women need counseling."

I have heard from countless women how they tried to address sexual concerns with their doctor and were told it was "normal aging" and how their significant other was given the answer to the same question with "try this [Viagra, Cialis, etc.]." Their concerns over vaginal dryness, discomfort with sex, less sensitivity, less arousal, less sexual frequency, and less sexual health were met with "you are getting old," while the health-care bias for men says we should treat erectile dysfunction as a vital part of humanity.

When women have an opportunity to experience sexuality the way they feel they could, the difference is quite remarkable. In addition to the two treatments I mentioned earlier—the nonsurgical laser treatment for vaginal relaxation and the nonsurgical filler to improve G-spot sensitivity—we offer a minor nonsurgical procedure that enhances the blood flow to the clitoris and allows women to have more clitoral orgasms much more quickly and easily.

While these functional treatments help improve a woman's sexuality, testosterone is the driver, as it is associated with desire, sensitivity, fulfillment, fantasy, and frequency.

Testosterone for Sexual Function

I can tell you that, from over a decade in the practice of treating women with hormone deficiency, sexual life can matter at any age. The studies I review in this chapter demonstrate the bias that the medical community has against women's sexual health after peak fertility. But as a physician who treats women physically for sexual health and functionally for libido, desire, and satisfaction, I have witnessed firsthand the importance of this element of health in women's lives.

In September 2000, the *New England Journal of Medicine,* one of the "gold standard" medical journals, reported on a study of testosterone replacement and its effect on impaired sexual function. The study looked at testosterone applied through the skin in women whose ovaries and uterus had been removed because of medical conditions. Again, a woman's ovaries produce about half of her testosterone; the rest comes from the adrenal glands, which are located above the kidneys. The women had been on HRT with an estrogen and synthetic progestin. The therapy was intended to reduce menopause symptoms such as hot flashes and night sweats, but the women felt that their libido and sense of well-being were also impaired by the ovary-removal surgery.

These were healthy women who had been in stable, monogamous, heterosexual relationships for at least a year. They were asked three questions:

1. At any time before surgery, would you have characterized your sex life as active and satisfying?

2. Since your surgery, has your sex life become less active and satisfying?

3. Would you prefer your sex life to be more active or more satisfying than it is now?

The study was a "crossover," meaning the subjects were switched between placebo and active testosterone, which is designed to reduce bias. The twelve-week study involved wearing a testosterone patch for two weeks, followed by a placebo patch for two weeks. There were two groups in the study. One group wore a standard dose (150 mg) of testosterone, the other group wore a double dose (300 mg). Sixty-five of the seventy-five enrolled women completed the study.

Desirous thoughts, frequency of sexual activity, and degree of pleasure and orgasm directly correlated to the dosage. While placebo wearers had the lowest sexual pleasure and activity, those wearing patches of 150 mg or 300 mg had better results, experiencing a doubling of the likelihood of having sex, having a sexual fantasy, or masturbating at least once a week. They didn't become sex-driven animals, but as women who had identified themselves as wanting more sex and sexual desires, they were happy to achieve improved sexual thoughts, arousal, frequency of sexual activity, initiation of sex, and orgasms. Satisfaction with their relationships improved as well. They had similar improvement in vitality and positive well-being, and they had less anxiety and fewer depressive moods.

There were no significant side effects, including no additional acne or facial hair growth, which are often assumed to occur with testosterone but are not a concern at therapeutic levels. Although it's true that women can grow muscle and exhibit masculine characteristics, that most often occurs with female bodybuilders who are purposely taking high doses of anabolic steroids to unnaturally build mass, not with women seeking to replenish normal testosterone levels.

Another study, conducted in 2003, included premenopausal women, ages thirty to forty-five, who were still having periods but self-reported diminished sexuality by rating the following:

- libido
- sexual activity
- satisfaction
- experience of pleasure
- sexual fantasy
- orgasm capacity

- relevance of sexuality in one's life

The women were healthy, lacked significant relationship problems, and were not on drugs that affected sexuality. Whether or not they were on birth control was irrelevant; however, women planning to get pregnant were not included in the study.

This study was also a twelve-week crossover; the women were treated with either placebo, low-dose testosterone, or higher-dose testosterone for six weeks and then switched to one of the other treatments. The study was also double blind—neither the participants nor the investigators knew what was in the vehicle administered, which in this case was a cream.

When comparing the testosterone group to the women in the placebo group, significant improvements were seen in psychological well-being and on the sexual scale. The higher dose of testosterone worked better than the lower dose. Once again, there were no issues with hair growth or acne, nor were there any other serious, adverse effects.

These two studies showed that testosterone, when taken alone or in addition to birth-control pills or standard drug HRT, improved sexuality in women.

A later study, conducted in 2015, took a closer look at testosterone dosage. This study involved women, ages twenty-one to sixty, who had undergone hysterectomies with or without ovary removal.

For twelve weeks prior to the start of the intervention, the women were placed on an estrogen patch, which is a common practice after a hysterectomy. They were given weekly shots of a placebo or of testosterone in four different dosages: 3 mg, 6.25 mg, 12.5 mg, or 25 mg. The women experienced improvements in sexual thoughts and desires, and in the group receiving the 25 mg dose, they also experienced an increase in frequency of sexual activity. Again, the general well-being scores increased relative to the doses of testosterone, demonstrating that proper dosage is also critical in testosterone replacement.

We have followed a similar approach in my practice. We used to administer a fairly low dose of testosterone for women in perimenopause or menopause. As time went on, we began increasing the dose of testosterone relative to estrogen based on newer clinical evidence, and our patients saw improvements as a result. Their mood and sexuality improved, as did all their menopause symptoms—at a far better rate than with the lower dosing.

What we discovered was that our patients were taking more than our recommended dose of testosterone because of the clear benefits they were seeing. It took some time for us to realize we were underdosing this hormone.

Today, for menopause, we predominantly use testosterone alone or along with tiny doses of estrogen. While this is a more modern approach, it is exactly what young, healthy ovaries did in the first place—testosterone pellets implanted in the skin almost perfectly mimic what happens in a young woman's body. We find that with testosterone alone, about 90 percent of women have relief of all menopause symptoms along with improvements of sexuality (such as lubrication, desire, and satisfaction). Some women, particularly those in the early stages of menopause or those already on an estrogen, need estrogen as well, but only for a short time.

A study in the early 1980s that was ahead of its time evaluated women who were on horse-based estrogen along with synthetic progestin. These women still had menopause symptoms—depression, sleep disturbance, palpitations, headaches, hot flashes—but the study was primarily aimed at addressing their low libido in spite of HRT.

The study administered 100 mg of testosterone and 40 mg of estrogen in pellet form. Today, we use a slightly higher dose of testosterone and a lower dose of estrogen because healthy young women have five to twenty times more testosterone than estrogen and can make their own estrogen from testosterone.

Before receiving the testosterone and estrogen pellets, 56 percent of women in the study reported their enjoyment of sex at nil, two-thirds had no orgasms for several months, and 90 percent never initiated sex with their partner. Within three months after the therapy, the women noticed improvements in all aspects of sexual symptoms. Again, this was a study conducted in the 1980s and confirmed even back then that testosterone enhanced sexuality in women.

We find that with the current recommendations—using testosterone as the primary hormone in menopause and estrogen as the "when-needed" hormone—the majority of women see improvement of their sexual health to a point where they are satisfied.

• •

Erika: Self-Esteem Saved

As an inside sales manager for a major equipment manufacturer, Erika needed to be on her game—on and off the job. But when she reached perimenopause, she found herself unexpectedly slowing down. Not only did she lack energy (in part from the many sleepless nights that had begun to creep into her world), but she also started experiencing night sweats, and she became moody and emotional—an obvious detriment to someone whose job involved working with customers all day. "I was tired most of the day and very irritable," Erika said.

Erika was already seeing Dr. Mok and team for other services when she heard about pellet hormones. "After I did some research on the pellet, I decided to ask Dr. Mok if I was a candidate for the treatment," she said. Erika said she asked a lot of questions during her discussion with Dr. Mok about the treatment, and then her blood work helped determine that she was a candidate.

On her next visit, Erika had pellets implanted, and the change was remarkable. "The treatment saved my self-esteem, my overall well-being, and probably even my marriage!" she said, adding how much she appreciated the calming, accommodating Allure team. "This has truly been a life-changing experience. I would recommend this for all women going through perimenopause. Why suffer when you don't have to?"

• •

In the 1980s, the data showed that testosterone was an integral part of women's health. But those findings fell to the wayside for a couple of decades until more recent research showed the vital importance of this hormone to women's sexual health and to overall well-being and health.

• •

The HRT Evolution

1940s HRT: Horse estrogen alone.

1970s HRT: Horse estrogen plus progesterone—worked well and reduced uterine cancer.

1980s HRT: Horse estrogen plus synthetic progestin. It became standard to prescribe HRT for most women in menopause, particularly for cardiac prevention.

1990s HRT: Horse estrogen is the number-one drug prescribed in the US for next two decades.

2002s HRT: Increased risk of breast cancer in women taking horse estrogen with synthetic progestin. HRT prescriptions drop precipitously.

2010s HRT: Greater than 50 percent reduction in risk of breast cancer and reduction of all menopause symptoms in women taking testosterone. Very little need for estrogen.

• •

The aforementioned studies demonstrate that sexual satisfaction can be successfully managed with testosterone replacement. The next two studies look at the link between hormone levels and sexual function and address the fact that testosterone and other androgens in the blood can be measured to see if blood hormone levels correspond to sexual health.

In 2002, a study looked at the link between testosterone levels and other androgens in relation to libido. The women in the study ranged in age from twenty-four to seventy-one years, and about half were in menopause. Each of the women reported a decrease in sexual desire, although they were all in stable relationships and did not have any medical or identifiable reason for a low sex drive. The women in menopause were on a standard HRT of estrogen plus a progestin, although some who had undergone a hysterectomy were on estrogen only because the progestin was designed to protect the uterus from estrogen growth.

The study's questionnaire asked the women to rate the following:

- arousal
- lubrication

- orgasm
- satisfaction
- pain

The control group consisted of women who reported no problems with sexual desire or activity.

In this study, total testosterone, free testosterone, and DHEA-S were depleted in all women complaining of sexual problems, compared to age-matched controls. There was a specific correlation between low testosterone and sexual dysfunction and between normal testosterone and normal sexual function.

Data reported in 2014 from a 3,302-participant study known as the Study of Women's Health Across the Nation (SWAN) identified sexual function as being important to 75 percent of the midlife women surveyed.

Participants reported on five factors of sexual activity: desire, arousal, orgasm, masturbation, and pain during intercourse (which of course can lead to sexual dysfunction).

Of these, sexual desire, arousal, and frequency of masturbation were positively associated with testosterone levels. The higher the level of testosterone, the more frequently sexual desire, sexual arousal, and masturbation occurred. Inversely, the lower the testosterone level, the lower the frequency of each of these. Pain, it turned out, was not correlated to any hormone studied.

In looking at other hormones, estrogen and SHBG had no relationship to any of the factors. However, follicle-stimulating hormone (FSH) typically followed the opposite pattern of testosterone; this is a predictable pattern because FSH rises when hormone production falls. Arousal, orgasm, and masturbation were negatively associated with FSH.

The results were mostly symptom based, but trends emerged: Low normal was more likely to be associated with sexual dysfunction. High normal was associated with better sexual function.

When we evaluate patients in our practice, we ask the same key questions as in these studies. Again, we know that sexuality can be a key component to women's health and quality of life.

Drugs versus Natural Therapies

For a time, the buzz in women's sexual health was about the drug I mentioned earlier, Addyi (flibanserin), which is touted as the "female Viagra." It isn't like Viagra at all, but it is an oral pill taken to increase sexual desire. Since the drug quite frankly doesn't do much for a woman's sexuality, it failed to reach the media frenzy that Viagra achieved when it hit the market.

Addyi doesn't increase orgasm, sensation, and pleasure the way testosterone replacement does. In fact, if you take the pill for an entire month, you will likely have 0.5 times more sexual encounters every month versus not taking it. That means sex one more time, every other month. Side effects include a risk of severe low blood pressure and loss of consciousness if you drink alcohol—a common beverage that can lead to sexual activity—or if you take over-the-counter cold medicines or supplements. Unlike hormones, which have virtually no side effects, with Addyi, women can experience dizziness, nausea, and increased sleepiness—maybe the increased sleepiness is the reason sex is so nominally increased?

Viagra (for men) was a media hit. Everyone has heard of it. Meanwhile, Addyi (for women) made barely a ripple. Was this an example of gender bias? No. Viagra worked. If a man has no erection, then intercourse is not going to happen. If a man takes Viagra, he may very well initiate sexual interaction regardless of libido or desire, since Viagra definitely helps a man achieve an erection within an hour or so. For women, desire, lubrication, sensation, and interest all play a role, but Addyi only sort of helps with interest—and then only every other month, when taken regularly.

Testosterone is clearly superior to and safer than the FDA-approved drug Addyi (flibanserin). So why aren't we hearing more about testosterone and women's sexual health? It's all about timing and the medical community's slow response and frustrating inability to face facts.

Back in 2005, when the North American Menopause Society released its position statement, it was clear that testosterone was more or less the standard of care for women's sexual health. A flurry of other activity also occurred around that time. In 2006, the Endocrine Society published clinical guidelines that stated it had no "data to support the use of testosterone or DHEA in women" and that there was "no evidence for an androgen-deficiency syndrome."

There you have it. In one major publication, the *Journal of Clinical Endocrinology & Metabolism*, it was determined that the condition known as *androgen deficiency*, which leads to sexual dysfunction in women, didn't even exist. Prior to the release of the publication, androgen deficiency had been shown to successfully be treated with testosterone replacement in numerous studies over decades.

As I mentioned earlier in the chapter, the year prior, in 2004, the FDA advisory panel voted unanimously not to approve the testosterone patch, the first and only drug to enhance a woman's sex drive, because of lack of evidence of long-term safety. The *New York Times* article reporting on the FDA vote quoted a cardiologist on the panel as saying, "I don't want to expose several million American women to the risk of heart attack and stroke" in order to have more sexual experiences. He was right when he identified that millions of

American women would want it, but he was wrong when he said it would expose women to risk of heart attack and stroke (those risks go down, as we will discuss in a subsequent chapter).

Sexuality in women was not perceived as having sufficient value, and even though the drug company pursuing approval of the patch had demonstrated that it was safe, it failed to prove that it wouldn't increase the risk of breast cancer or other disease, in spite of decades of research and an abundance of literature that demonstrated testosterone's safety and its protective effects against breast cancer.

At the time, Proctor & Gamble was seeking FDA approval for testosterone to improve sexual desire in women who had their uterus and ovaries removed from a hysterectomy, and there was also a concern that other women would want to use it as well. By law, the FDA approves a drug for a specific condition, and then doctors can choose to use the same drug for a nonapproved use; drug companies have to define a very narrow range of people to study the use of a drug on, and then logic and practice of medicine can dictate how it is eventually used. So the fear was that women who had not had their ovaries removed would want to have sex more often, even though the company was trying to get it approved for women without ovaries.

When the FDA evaluates a drug, one part of the approval process involves a committee deciding whether something is "clinically meaningful." About 25 percent of the advisory panel looking at the Proctor & Gamble testosterone felt that women wanting more sex and achieving sexual pleasure and orgasm more often had no clinically meaningful significance.

I want to make this clear: some FDA advisory panelists felt that women's sexual health had no meaningful clinical significance. Sexuality may not be the number-one concern of every woman, but it does have significance. As a doctor treating tens of thousands of women, I can tell you that the panel was dead wrong, and if you are reading this book, I am sure you will agree.

A Frustrating Journey

As you may see by now, getting testosterone approved to treat female sexual dysfunction has been something of a frustrating journey, compounded by the absurd debate between medical societies as to whether sexual dysfunction even occurs in women. Here's a timeline of some of the significant milestones:

1980–1990s: Low testosterone in women is shown to be linked to less sexual health, and clinical studies show sexual pleasure, desire, frequency, and satisfaction are improved with testosterone replacement.

2003: Proctor & Gamble's attempts to get approval for a testosterone treatment are denied by the FDA unanimously because of inadequate long-term studies, even though there had been abundant research demonstrating safety. One of the panel members states that having sex more often is not important, and the many members feel that decreased sexuality has no clinical meaningfulness.

2005: Policy statement from the North American Menopause Society recommends use of testosterone for sexual health for a variety of reasons and cites safety and clinical meaningfulness.

2006: The Endocrine Society denies that androgen deficiency exists and states that testosterone doesn't work in spite of overwhelming evidence to the contrary. A separate endocrine group, the American Association of Clinical Endocrinologists, had urged FDA committee approval of the testosterone drug three years earlier.

Watchdog and advocacy groups join the argument against FDA approval of testosterone to improve sexual function for women with their ovaries surgically removed because "it would probably be used by women of various ages." The groups were concerned that women in perimenopause and menopause who had not had their ovaries removed would want to have more sexual desire and pleasure and would use testosterone if it was approved as a drug.

2014: The Endocrine Society makes a new clinical practice guideline based on this conclusion: "We continue to recommend against making the diagnosis of androgen deficiency syndrome in healthy women because there is a lack of a well-defined syndrome, and data correlating androgen levels with specific signs or symptoms are unavailable." This comes after endocrinology groups express intent to get FDA testosterone approval for women for sexual health, the North American Menopause Society position statement, and the publishing of numerous clinical studies that tie androgen levels to sexual health. It is quite unusual for a medical society to make such a biased statement, but there is a clear pattern of political argument among the medical societies.

The Endocrine Society's use of phrasing such as "specific signs and symptoms" is factually correct, as sexual issues such as desire, orgasm, fantasies, and pleasure are not specific and cannot be proven to a third party. Yet things like pain and mood are considered specific signs and symptoms, and clinicians rely on patients' statements rather than having scientific proof of those factors.

The Endocrine Society recommends against routine testing of testosterone in women with sexual dysfunction because such dysfunction can be caused by things other than low testosterone. Their suggestion to not conduct tests would equate to negligence in any other field of medicine. The society agreed that evidence supports the use of testosterone treatment for postmenopausal women with sexual dysfunction due to hypoactive desire disorder but noted that testosterone preparations for women are not available in many countries, including the United States. That latter statement is also incorrect because testosterone preparations for women have been available at pharmacies and made in FDA-approved labs for years.

In reality, the FDA has a specific exemption for products such as testosterone. FDA approval is typically thought of when we talk about new drugs that are invented. But some compounds, such as hormones, do not require FDA approval because they are hormones, not drugs, and already widely available and prepared by pharmacists. For this, there is a separate approval-process form (503B), which allows a smaller manufacturer to produce a drug that is already in the public domain, providing it passes FDA inspection and follows standard safety protocols. That's how a number of well-established drugs have been made available to the public without a new indication or the financial backing of large pharmaceutical companies. In our practice, we use testosterone from manufacturers that are registered under this special FDA 503B section.

The Endocrine Society's guidelines also recommended testosterone use only after menopause, which also runs contrary to science. Menopause is an abrupt decrease in fertility and estrogen and progesterone production. Testosterone drop-off is much more insidious and not tied to menopause. It is as if the Endocrine Society, which represents specialists in hormones, is ignoring the physiology of menopause and hormone production. Their bias against women's sexuality has forced them to ignore well-established scientific facts.

The Endocrine Society also noted that "government agency-approved and monitored dose-appropriate preparations are not widely available." Their opposition was to the perceived lack of government-monitored dosage. Medical societies are becoming more and more political and trying to control government oversight of relationships between physicians and their patients. The government does approve and monitor the manufacturers of testosterone for women, and the society suggests that the government, not the physician, determines the proper dosage for individual women.

A more absurd part of the guideline reads, "We recommend against routine treatment of women with low androgen levels due to . . . oophorectomy, or other conditions associated with low androgen levels because of lack of adequate data supporting efficacy and/or long term safety." Although the Endocrine Society acknowledges that both oophorectomy (removal of the ovaries) and hysterectomy result in markedly lower androgen levels, it is well-known that women who have undergone those procedures have more sexual health dysfunction. And while I agree with the phrasing "against routine treatment" (because any treatment should be made individually), again, the long-term safety of testosterone has been well established, so treating only a very select group of women for sexual-health reasons for a short period of time makes no sense.

The Endocrine Society's statement that testosterone blood level doesn't correlate well to symptoms is somewhat accurate. Treatment with testosterone should always be based more on symptoms than just a blood test. In my practice, we perform tests to confirm what we suspect, and if the blood test and symptoms do not correlate, we look for other causes.

The Endocrine Society, on the other hand, recommends that the testosterone level should be checked before treatment and frequently during therapy. This seems to be a contradictory statement: A major medical society is saying that a well-known condition doesn't really exist, that it cannot be measured or validated, and that there are no treatments available. Then they go on to say that if physicians do treat sexual dysfunction due to androgen deficiency, testosterone levels should be measured frequently. The whole position is absurd.

The same guidelines refute the findings of notable studies such as SWAN, and the guidelines more or less deem a woman's lack of sexual desire over time and want of more desire to be a "normal," common complaint and that poor relationships are a more likely reason for the problem. This would be equivalent to saying that high blood pressure can be a normal fact of life as people age, so we should not measure or treat it.

In short, the 2014 Endocrine Society guidelines are fraught with contradictions, ignore science, and suffer from member bias. This is just one piece of evidence of how medical societies have completely misinterpreted clearly established facts and are totally out of touch with the needs of women today.

• •

The Winning Edge

- Testosterone is a proven treatment for sexual health in women.
- There has been amazing resistance by the medical community toward women's sexuality.
- Testosterone has been shown to safely improve a womans sexual desire, arousal, sensitivy, frequency of orgasms and fantasies in women who desire this in their lives.
- Testosterone is in a class of hormones called androgens, which men and women both have.
- Medical societies have denied that androgen deficiency exists in spite of evidence to the contrary.
- A position statement by the North American Menopause Society supported use of testosterone therapy for postmenopausal women with decreased sexual desires.
- Several studies demonstrate that sexual satisfaction can be successfully managed with testosterone replacement.
- Testosterone is clearly superior and safer than the FDA-approved drug flibanserin or any other known treatment.
- Medical societies can be contradictory and ignore science and suffer from gender bias.

• •

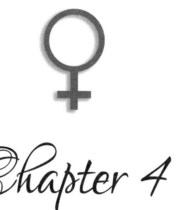

Chapter 4

CARDIOVASCULAR HEALTH: HORMONES AND THE SYNTHETIC PROGESTIN CONNECTION

The fear that occurred from observations of the negative effects of synthetic hormones on the cardiovascular system should not apply to natural hormone replacement. In fact, long-term use of *natural* hormones in menopause reduces a woman's chance of dying of a heart attack by over 70 percent!

Heart disease is the top cause of death for women in the United States, followed by cancer—lung, breast, ovarian, cervical, ovarian, in that order—then stroke, chronic obstructive lung disease (including emphysema), and pneumonia/influenza.

While not as emotionally charged a topic as breast cancer, heart disease is about ten times more likely than breast cancer to cause death in a woman. As a patient, it's important that you have a very clear understanding when deciding whether to accept or decline modern HRT.

While HRT has for decades been used routinely to help women relieve postmenopausal symptoms—hot flashes, night sweats, sleep disturbance, and the like—in 1987, the NIH undertook a major study to determine if HRT could also protect the heart and cardiovascular system.

The Postmenopausal Estrogen/Progestin study (PEPI), which looked at therapy using estrogen or estrogen plus synthetic progestin, was a landmark study that stimulated a change in the practice of medicine.

Because prior evidence suggested that hormones provided heart protection, the government sponsored a larger study with the intention of advising doctors and women. The PEPI study initially found that HRT offered protection against heart disease to women in menopause. The study's recommendations were to initiate HRT at the onset of menopause for cardiovascular protection and improved quality of life.

Unfortunately, the health-care community later reversed its recommendations for HRT for cardioprotection due to later flawed studies and misinterpreted data—even when the data was correct.

The evidence regarding hormones and cardioprotection has been mounting. Briefly, hormones are cardioprotective, but synthetic progestin is not and may even be harmful to some aspects of women's health.

In this chapter, I'll show how testosterone is connected to a woman's cardiac system. I'll also review the scientific literature from a historical standpoint up to the present day, and I'll share with you how emerging evidence influenced the practice of medicine.

Then and Now

In the 1980s and 1990s, studies suggested that it was more or less the standard of care to use HRT to reduce a woman's risk of developing heart disease. Studies showed that as a woman's estrogen declined, her risk of cardiac disease increased, but that HRT could reverse that trend.

The practice of using HRT to reduce heart disease had actually started some years earlier. Between 1960 and 1975, the rate of prescribed estrogen replacement for women in menopause shot through the roof. Publicized data, news articles, and books proclaimed estrogen to be an elixir to help women through menopause.

In 1975, reports surfaced that estrogen replacement led to an increase in endometrial cancer. That led to a tapering off of estrogen for a few years until it was clarified that another hormone, namely progesterone, was needed to avoid stimulating the uterus. When progesterone (or later, synthetic progestin) was added to estrogen, the risk of endometrial cancer was negated.

That led to a rise in HRT prescriptions again, and Premarin, or horse estrogen, became the most common drug prescription in the United States, a position it held through the next couple of decades.

In the late 1990s, the results of the PEPI study were published after a decade-long investigation. The study was conducted by the NIH and the National Heart, Lung, and Blood Institute.

The aim of the PEPI study was to determine whether the common practice of prescribing HRT for women entering menopause and staying on HRT for life was appropriate.

The PEPI study included one placebo group and four treatment groups: one estrogen-only group; two estrogen-plus-synthetic-progestin groups, one of which took the drugs daily and another that took the drugs twelve days a month; and a group that took estrogen plus natural progesterone. All of the women were in menopause, and the women in the estrogen-only group had no uterus.

PEPI Study Results

- Estrogen alone raises HDL (good cholesterol).
- Estrogen plus progesterone or progestin protected the lining of the uterus from overgrowth.
- Estrogen plus synthetic progestin raised HDL, but not as much as estrogen plus natural progesterone or estrogen alone.
- All regimens nearly equally reduced LDL (bad cholesterol).
- Fibrinogen levels decreased. High fibrinogen levels are linked to stroke and heart attack.
- Blood pressure was not altered.
- No other significant changes were noted.

The intent of the PEPI study was to follow the women for years longer to assess long-term outcomes, but the major guidance was that women should consider HRT after menopause not only for symptom relief but also for cardiac protection. It was also found that natural progesterone was preferable to synthetic progestin.

As a result of the PEPI study, prescribing habits changed. There had been no doubt that hormone replacement improved quality of life for women in menopause, but now there was evidence that even for women with few menopause symptoms or little distress, hormone replacement should be considered to protect the heart.

Then came the much-publicized WHI clinical trials, which changed HRT habits substantially for years. I discussed these in chapter 1, but to recap, one of the trials in the ten-year study was stopped because statistical evidence found an increase of breast cancer of 8/10,000 person-years, and a 7/10,000 person-years increase in coronary heart disease. The study used Premarin, which is a CEE (horse estrogens); Provera (medroxyprogesterone acetate), a synthetic progestin; and Prempro, a combination of both.

After the WHI study, use of HRT fell by 50 percent across the country. As there had been extensive studies at the same time as the WHI study that showed safety when actual hormones (not synthetic drugs) were used, physicians such as myself became more engaged in taking women off of synthetic hormone drugs and changing them over to natural hormone replacement.

Two major differences between the PEPI study and the WHI trials were the inclusion or exclusion of natural progesterone, along with the timing as to when the drugs were administered. While the PEPI study more or less mimicked what was happening at the time in US health care (starting women on HRT at the onset of menopause), the WHI trials started women on HRT when they were much older and well into menopause. The PEPI study, therefore, focused more on prevention, while the WHI trials added the treatment later on. This major flaw in the interpretation of the WHI study was more clearly realized well after the much-publicized results were reported and distributed, and the interpretation, in spite of its flaws, has had a major, negative impact on women's health ever since. Doctors reduced prescriptions of all hormone preparations that have been solidly proven to reduce symptoms, improve quality of life, and be cardioprotective because of the results of a largely flawed interpretation of a drug trial. The trial itself was not flawed in design; it was actually a very elegant study. But the interpretation was flawed, as the study was examining a specific drug used in a fashion that did not mimic the current practice of medicine.

New Opinion Statement

In June 2013, the American College of Obstetricians and Gynecologists published a committee opinion regarding estrogen and progestin (synthetic progestin). The American College of Obstetricians and Gynecologists' opinion was designed as a guideline for gynecologists, but other specialists tended to review it as well.

Here is a quick review of the types of hormones:

- Estrogen is considered the dominant hormone in women, even though testosterone is about five to twenty times more abundant than estrogen in women.

- Estrogen is responsible for secondary female characteristics as girls grow into women and has a significant influence on female characteristics. It stimulates growth of the uterus lining, lubricates the vagina, and induces bone formation to help prevent osteoporosis.

- There are numerous subtypes of estrogens. There are three principal subtypes:

  ▫ Estradiol is a potent estrogen, considered to be the dominant estrogen in women. It is a true natural estrogen and is the most commonly used estrogen for menopause after Premarin. Estradiol is made from testosterone or other androgens through a process called aromatization. Medically, estradiol is known as E2.

  ▫ Estrone is less common and less potent than estradiol. It is aromatized from testosterone in the fat cells and in the gut. There are several subtypes of estrone that have a fairly clear link to breast cancer and other disease, and it is postulated that this is part of the reason that obesity is linked to breast cancer and other disorders. More fat cells can make more of the unhealthy estrone. Medically, estrone is known as E1.

▫ Estriol is not very potent. It is present in very high levels during pregnancy, hence the "pregnancy glow." It has significant positive effects on the skin and vaginal, as well as mucosal moisture. Medically, estriol is known as E3.

- Premarin is a conjugated equine estrogen (CEE) originally taken from the urine of a five-year-old pregnant horse. Today, Premarin is synthesized from soybeans in a way that represents the makeup of estrogens from a five-year-old pregnant horse.

- Synthetic progestin is designed specifically to protect the uterus from cancer when exposed to external estrogen. The uterine lining has progesterone receptors. The estrogen/progesterone ratios determine if the lining grows or sheds (a menstrual period). If the estrogen is unopposed by progesterone or a progestin drug, it can eventually turn the stimulated uterus lining into cancer.

The American College of Obstetricians and Gynecologists' opinion was to recommend against using estrogen and synthetic progestin for the sole purpose of cardiovascular health. Remember, thirty years earlier, it was recommended that women use HRT for prevention of heart protection. The opinion also addressed the "hormone haters" who had been trying to paint HRT as cardiotoxic. The formers of the opinion noted that large studies such as the notable WHI trials were flawed and that there was no evidence to suggest that HRT should be discontinued as women age for reasons of heart protection. The opinion identified that there was evidence that starting HRT early is heart protective but stated that should not be the only reason to start it. To summarize, they found that synthetic hormone replacement could be used for symptoms of menopause, shouldn't be used for the sole intent of cardiac protection, and shouldn't be discontinued for cardiac risk concerns. It was fairly noncommittal.

The Timing Effect

In the WHI trial, there was a small increase in cardiac events in women taking horse estrogen plus synthetic progestin, but as I mentioned earlier, it appeared to be a timing issue. When elderly women, potentially with preexisting heart disease, initiate HRT for the first time, there can be more cardiac events, and the WHI trial was based on that scenario. But when started younger and continued, there is the benefit of cardiac protection.

A pair of trials called Heart and Estrogen/Progestin Study (HERS) and HERSII focused on women with preexisting heart disease.

Women who start synthetic HRT at ages fifty to fifty-nine trend toward decreased mortality and cardiac disease. The women in the WHI trial started synthetic HRT at around sixty-three years, which led to a timing hypothesis on HRT—that starting HRT earlier conferred protection, while starting it ten years after menopause led to more nonfatal cardiac events. In other words, at an older age, HRT caused no deaths but more problems.

In the WHI trial that included women with hysterectomies who were on CEE but not on progestin, CT scans were performed on the heart to determine if vascular damage was occurring or was prevented with HRT. Women taking horse estrogen alone had a significant reduction in coronary artery calcification scores versus those women taking a placebo. In other words, women on horse estrogen plus progesterone had cardiac protection if therapy was started early. If they were on estrogen only, they not only had fewer heart attacks but the CT scan also showed they were significantly less likely to have one. But if they started horse estrogen and synthetic progestin a decade after menopause, there were more nonfatal cardiac events.

Other studies have shown that women with ovaries removed during a hysterectomy had better heart protection if they started estrogen right away; otherwise, they were more likely to develop heart plaques.

The American College of Obstetricians and Gynecologists noted that, even though some government-sponsored agencies have advised discontinuation of HRT after sixty-five and won't pay for it in some cases, they disagree because the assumption of health risks are false.

The American College of Obstetrics and Gynecology also recommends that progesterone may be more cardioprotective than synthetic progestin. It certainly is, and I'll review the progesterone connection again later.

The Danish Study

When taken long term, natural estrogen cuts heart attack deaths by 73 percent. That was the finding of a study published in 2010 in the *British Medical Journal*, which sought to clarify the questions posed by the WHI and HERS trials: When should HRT be started? Should it be used only for menopausal symptoms, or can it be used to protect the heart? Does it cause heart attacks or prevent them? Again, the WHI and HERS trials were potentially flawed in that they did not replicate the current practice of medicine (to start hormones early in menopause and continue them for years). Additionally, they did not did they evaluate the use of human-based hormones, but only synthetically manufactured drugs.

The Danish study enrolled more than two thousand women, with half of them on HRT and the other half on a placebo. The study was carried out for eleven years, until it was stopped because of negative pressure from the larger WHI trial. But the researchers in the Danish study continued to follow the women for up to sixteen years.

The Danish study more closely followed what happens in the normal practice of medicine, which is to start women on HRT at menopause, rather than a decade later. The women were about forty-five to fifty-eight years old, and they had been in menopause for one to two years or had started in perimenopause.

Women with an intact uterus were put on estradiol (the human estrogen, not horse estrogen) and progestin (synthetic progestin). Women with hysterectomies were given estrogen alone.

Of significant note is that *deaths due to cardiovascular causes were reduced by 73 percent in the HRT group versus the placebo group.* Cardiac events (nonfatal) were decreased by over 50 percent. At the ten-year point of the Danish study, there were fewer deaths with HRT than with no HRT; in the WHI trials, the death rate was equal. When the Danish study tracked the women longer, up to sixteen years, the benefit of HRT on cardiac death and disease was profoundly different than in the WHI trial, which was flawed in regard to the timing of initiation of treatment.

So the Danish study showed that women who were treated in the conventional way—with human-type, natural estrogen administered at the onset of menopause—had a remarkable reduction in deaths.

Progesterone versus Synthetic Progestin

Progesterone is another protective hormone. Again, the synthetic form of progesterone is progestin, which is a drug made solely to protect the uterus from unopposed estrogen.

In 2000, the *Journal of the American College of Cardiology* reported on another study that contradicted the findings of the flawed HERS trials and showed that natural estrogen and natural progesterone improve cardiac performance by 100 percent in women with preexisting heart disease.

The study identified potential flaws in the HERS study and found that natural progesterone, not synthetic progestin, clearly improves cardiac profiles in postmenopausal women with heart disease. The study also acknowledged that estrogen is cardioprotective in virtually every model experimentally tested and that estrogen seems to be anti-atherogenic, meaning it helps prevent the buildup of plaques in the arteries.

Furthermore, the 2000 study found that synthetic progestin blocks the protective nature of estrogen—indeed, the intent of the study was to determine if the very nature of using a totally synthetic progestin rather than a natural progesterone undermined the protective effects of progesterone on the cardiovascular system.

This landmark study enrolled women with at least 70 percent narrowing of a coronary artery, which is a major risk factor for dying of a heart attack. It was a crossover study, so participants took estradiol and either a synthetic progestin or naturally produced progesterone, and they flipped between the two to eliminate bias. The women underwent stress tests to determine the amount of time it took to begin cardiac stress.

When the study started, the women were on estrogen alone. In the stress test, the time to cardiac stress increased somewhat.

When they were put on estrogen plus progesterone, the time until changes recorded on the EKG almost doubled.

When the women were on estrogen plus progestin, the time to heart ischemia was much faster—about half the time.

So the take-home point is that estrogen improved cardiac performance. Adding a synthetic worsened cardiac performance, which occurred in prior studies. But estrogen plus natural progesterone improved cardiac performance by about 100 percent. Currently, there remains a bias against treating women with risk factors for heart disease or with preexisting heart disease because of the negative effects of synthetic hormone drugs. It is critical for patients and doctors to understand that natural hormone replacement is not only safe but also reduces the rate of a fatal heart attack by 73 percent and improves cardiac performance by 100 percent.

In our practice, we use natural hormones for women with cardiac risk. In my opinion, it is mandatory. To my knowledge, there are no other studies with any drug showing such a profound improvement.

Route of Administration

It's important to note that the form of administration affects the efficacy of the hormone administered. The superior delivery system for hormones available today is the pellet.

A hormone pellet is a compressed, rice-sized medication delivery system. It is placed under the skin through a tiny incision and slowly breaks down and releases the hormone over a few months. The benefits of the pellets are that the levels of hormone delivered are extremely consistent; the hormone bypasses your liver, so you don't need to take a mega-dose like with a pill; and you don't even have to remember to take it.

A study on women with prior hysterectomy conducted at the department of obstetrics and gynecology at the University of California, Los Angeles, compared an estrogen skin patch applied every three to four days to pellet estrogen inserted once.

In the patch group, the blood hormone level peaked in about four hours and then tapered off to about half its original level between eight hours up to the three-day duration of the patch. The pellet peaked at twenty-four hours and remained essentially unchanged for the same three-day period. The pellet also stayed stable for the thirty-two-week study period.

The patch group's blood estrogen levels varied from a 25 percent increase to a 225 percent increase over the study period. The pellet group had no significant fluctuation.

In the group with the patch, there was no significant change on HDL cholesterol, whereas the pellet had a beneficial effect on HDL and on cholesterol-to-HDL ratio.

The pellet is superior not only for avoiding the first-pass effect from the liver and driving down inflammation and SHBG absorption but also for cost and convenience. When estrogen is taken as a pill, a dose approximately a hundred thousand times greater than needed is used because of how it is absorbed. As I mentioned earlier, when the pill is swallowed, the liver senses that you have eaten estrogen and makes SHBG to bind to the estrogen that you have ingested. But SHBG also binds other beneficial hormones and is linked to inflammation. Patches or topical creams do not have this response with SHBG but do lead to substantial peaks and valleys in hormone levels throughout the day or period used. Pellets are superior in not only the lack of lowering other beneficial hormone levels but also in providing extremely steady hormone levels—the way the ovaries performed when they were functioning.

The Testosterone Connection

As I mentioned earlier, testosterone is a more accurate predictor of heart disease than cholesterol and other lipids. Women with low testosterone have more heart disease, and women with normal or higher testosterone have less heart disease.

There is a general bias or fear that since testosterone is more prevalent in men than women, and men have heart disease typically ten years younger than women, then maybe testosterone causes heart disease. That is incorrect. For men, the data clearly supports that testosterone replacement is beneficial for symptoms of low testosterone and protects against obesity, metabolic syndrome, heart disease, and death.

In comparison, let's look at how this mostly forgotten, dominant hormone affects women's cardiovascular health. It has been observed that postmenopausal women with extreme levels of sex hormones were more likely to suffer heart disease. But keep in mind, these are extremes. Why is the estrogen extremely low or the testosterone extremely high? Because these women have confounding health issues leading to extreme changes. That does not imply causation.

In 2014, Harvard, Brigham and Women's Hospital in Boston, and Boston Medical Center published a study to address the theory that the extremely high levels of sex hormones in insulin resistance syndrome, obesity, and polycystic ovarian syndrome may not be causes of heart disease but may instead be a response to the numerous other factors associated with those diseases.

The study enrolled women who had undergone a hysterectomy. All women were given an estradiol patch and injections of a placebo or various doses of testosterone.

The researchers performed various tests and assays to see if there was a link between elevating testosterone and the conditions seen in people with abnormally high testosterone levels. In other words, does high testosterone in a subgroup of women cause obesity, insulin resistance, and polycystic ovary syndrome? Or do those conditions wreak havoc on hormone levels?

The study showed that no dose of testosterone caused insulin resistance, obesity, or negative cardiovascular events.

Another study published in 2000 in *Heart, Lung and Circulation* reported the results of adding testosterone to women already on estrogen. The researchers added rice-sized testosterone pellets to the participants' HRT regimen. They measured various markers of vascular endothelium (lining of the blood vessel wall), blood flow, and inflammation. They found that the addition of testosterone pellets both improved the flow of blood and relaxed the wall of the vessel—both positive effects on the cardiovascular system.

Earlier, I discussed how women with various diseases and extremely altered estrogen and testosterone levels had more cardiovascular risk factors and events. I also discussed how it is the disease that alters the hormones, not the hormones themselves that cause the disease. But what about women who are not in a chronic disease state with extreme hormone levels?

That question was explored by a study published in 2003 in the *International Journal of Cardiology*. Armed with plenty of data showing that low testosterone in men is associated with premature heart disease and that supplementation of testosterone in men with heart disease was cardioprotective, researchers set out to measure nonextreme hormone levels of testosterone in women and correlate them to the risk of cardiac disease.

The study group was composed of women undergoing coronary angioplasty for diagnostic reasons. These were women in menopause who didn't know if they had heart disease or not and were getting a test to check.

The women with angiographically proven coronary artery disease had a tendency for unfavorable lipid levels, as predicted.

But researchers also found another consistent pattern. Women with normal or high testosterone levels tended to have perfectly normal hearts, and women with low testosterone tended to have coronary artery disease.

There was a strong correlation between low testosterone in women and coronary artery disease, while the lipids had only a moderate correlation. Yet again, we see that low testosterone is a more accurate predictor of heart disease than high cholesterol.

Another study done at Johns Hopkins and published in 2002 evaluated postmenopausal hormone level and the relative risk of atherosclerosis. Atherosclerosis is the most common cardiovascular disease, and there are various ways to measure it.

One very sensitive and specific way to measure whole body atherosclerosis with a simple mechanism is by measuring the thickness of the wall of the carotid artery. The carotid is located just below the skin in the neck, which is in the perfect place to measure with ultrasound. It's the site where the pulse is typically measured.

The study looked at fifteen thousand people, both men and women, who had scans at one, two, and three years.

Those with identifiable disease were the study group, and those with normal arteries were the control group.

Study group patients, as expected, were more likely than the control group to smoke, trended toward worse lipid profiles, and had higher blood pressures, more insulin resistance, and lower HDL (good cholesterol).

Women with the highest level of estrone, the unfavorable estrogen, had the most cardiovascular disease.

The women with the highest testosterone levels tended to have normal arteries, while women with the lowest testosterone had the most atherosclerosis.

So unlike the "extremely high" testosterone found in certain disease states, higher testosterone in women is associated with less cardiovascular disease.

• •

The Winning Edge

- Hormone replacement not only improves symptoms of menopause and quality of life but also can protect your heart.
- Women with preexisting heart disease see a 100 percent improvement of cardiac function with natural hormone replacement.
- There are many options for administration, from pills to creams to implants, as well as options of using synthetic drugs or actual hormones.
- Science has shown us that women who initiate hormones at the onset of menopause or perimenopause will have less heart disease and a risk reduction of 73 percent in death from heart attack.
- Taking hormone replacement that mimics as closely as possible what nature provided prior to menopause is the safest, most natural, and most protective option.
- Menopause occurs when the ovaries are removed surgically or when they fail naturally over time. The dominant

hormone in young, healthy women is testosterone, and low testosterone in women is a strong predictor of heart disease.

- Tiny hormone pellets placed just under the skin give the most consistent and reliable blood levels of hormones and most closely mimic nature.

• •

Chapter 5

THE THIRD CAUSE OF OBESITY
AND THE LINK TO HORMONES

The number-one concern I hear from women entering menopause is about the weight gain. While the biggest discovery in the history of weight gain and obesity was made recently, most people haven't heard anything about it yet.

As I've mentioned in previous chapters, when women age, their hormone levels decline. With declining hormone levels, women become not only symptomatic of menopause but also more rapidly develop signs of what is commonly referred to as "normal aging." While youthful hormone levels (particularly testosterone) reduce breast cancer, protect the heart, and improve sexuality, there is also evidence that declining hormones have a dramatic impact on weight.

The costs of weight gain and obesity are substantial, for both the individual and for public health in general. With weight gain, heart disease, diabetes, cancer, hypertension, and other serious disorders increase in frequency.

Again, menopause is caused by ovarian failure or removal. But a number of studies have shown that while ovarian failure leads to weight gain, ovarian preservation is linked to favorable weight maintenance. There are also studies that show how maintaining healthy hormone levels with hormone supplementation can lead to better weight management into menopause.

I've been talking about the bias against hormone replacement on the part of medical societies. There is also a disconnect between many physicians and their patients, largely because misinformation in the media is making it difficult to discern fact from fiction. Much of that is because of very limited and flawed studies that catch the attention of news organizations and the media. Yet the lion's share of research that is published and shows the overwhelming safety of hormones for menopause is not as controversial and doesn't get the same attention. It takes years before trends in medicine change, in part because many doctors simply don't review the latest literature on a consistent and disciplined basis. And the misunderstanding of scientific data by the public-health community has meant that millions of women were taken off hormone replacement and subjected to unnecessarily increased risk of cancer and heart disease.

In my opinion, treating ovarian failure or removal with hormone replacement is like treating any other condition. If a patient presents with thyroid failure, no reasonable physician would be opposed to thyroid hormone replacement. If a woman developed high blood pressure, doctors would never suggest, "It's a normal part of life, live with it." So why do some doctors and their patients shun hormone replacement, viewing menopause as "normal aging"? Why do some women take pride in going through menopause "naturally," without help? While that may sound like a healthy option or a badge of courage, ultimately, it's not healthy.

Withholding hormone replacement for women in menopause is as absurd as withholding treatment for heart disease, diabetes, and hypertension.

The Impact of Microbiota—Gut Bacteria

Microbiota, or gut bacteria, and hormones are crucially linked, but before I dive into their relationship, I'd like to give some background information on the bacteria in our bodies. Someday, we will look back and realize that the discovery of the effect of microbiota on our health was one of the biggest discoveries of our lifetimes. Right now, we are just beginning to understand what this means.

The discovery of microbiota was possible through the ability to detect bacteria by mapping its DNA.

There are more than a hundred trillion bacteria in your body, largely concentrated in your colon. These bacteria are now found to be linked to various disease states such as autoimmune conditions, hypertension, diabetes, certain cancers, and obesity (or leanness). These bacteria are what I call "the third cause of obesity."

The first and second causes are quite clear: poor diet and lack of exercise. But the third cause of obesity has been extensively researched in the past decade, and this research has yielded some pretty amazing data.

Each person is an organism with a genetic code. It was long assumed that each person's genetic code had a predictor of obesity. However, as it turns out, there are also more than a hundred trillion microorganisms living in each person's gastrointestinal track, and these microorganisms each have their own DNA. The genetic strains of these microbiota can forecast, predict, or determine whether someone is normal weight, overweight, or obese. Someone who has a poor diet and doesn't exercise may still be very thin because of their own protective microbiota. This person's gut bacteria are very biodiverse, meaning that he or she has a very high number of varied species of bacteria and that those bacteria have hung around for most of that person's life.

In most people, however, microbiota can change from "good" to "bad" depending on what they're fed, their environment, to some degree the way different people are genetically programmed to respond to the bacteria, and the people they interact with (who may transfer bacteria like a cold). For most people, however, microbiota depends primarily on diet and exposures in our society.

Good bacteria in the gut break down food, passing on the nutrients and anti-inflammatory properties for the body to absorb and use. During the process of breaking the food down, the good bacteria digests a lot of calories, which keeps a person at a normal weight even when they cheat and consume too many calories. Bad bacteria, meanwhile, pass along toxins such as endotoxins and immunotoxins. Bad bacteria also help extract energy out of food, but they consume very few calories, which makes a person put on weight.

The discovery of microbiota is exciting because it has given us a better understanding of how we can transform from being an obese society to being a normal-weight society. No longer will we have the reputation of spreading "the fat bug" around the world, as I recently heard one British woman describe our situation.

The NIH notes that between 1962 and 1980, the rates of overweight, obese, and extremely obese Americans stayed pretty much the same. And the percentage of overweight adults hasn't changed much between 1962 and 2010.

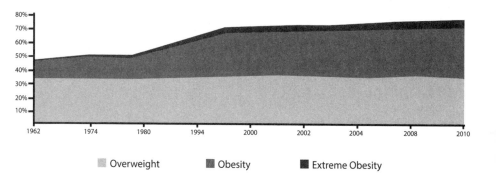

Overweight   Obesity   Extreme Obesity

But from 1980 to the late 1990s, the rates of obesity and extreme obesity skyrocketed, and those numbers have remained intact.

- **Overweight**—In 1962, 32 percent of adult Americans were overweight; in 2010, 34 percent of Americans were overweight. That's not much change.
- **Obese**—In 1962, 13 percent of American adults were obese. From the late 1990s to today, about 36 percent of Americans are obese. That represents nearly a tripling of the numbers.
- **Extremely obese**—From the late 1990s to today, extreme obesity went from 1 percent to 5 percent, a five-fold increase.

Studies looking at Americans activities and dietary changes cannot account for such a dramatic change in the rate of obesity. Yes, we eat more and exercise less, so the numbers of overweight adults went from 32 percent to 34 percent. But obesity and extreme obesity skyrocketed in the same time frame.

That's where understanding and managing microbiota, also called the *microbiome*, come into play—and where hormones can be instrumental.

Hormones and Weight

The most common complaint women have with menopause or hormone changes is weight gain. Increased fat storage, increased cholesterol, and decreased sensitivity to insulin are commonly seen. But hormone replacement combined with lifestyle changes can reverse this complaint, as demonstrated by the results of a 1999 study from Switzerland.

The study evaluated the effect of transdermal estrogen and an oral progesterone on weight in menopausal, overweight women. Every participant's bloodwork was evaluated, their weight was measured, and their baseline resting-calorie burn was assessed.

They were trained on proper eating habits for a month before the onset of the study. Then they were put on a meal plan of 35 percent fat, 50 percent carbohydrates, and 15 percent protein. Today, much higher percentages of protein are recommended, which is a metabolic mistake, as I'll discuss later.

The individuals in the study were followed for three months.

The members of the control group, who took only a placebo, experienced no weight loss, even though they were placed on a strict and healthy diet.

Women in the treatment group, who received topical estrogen, were on the same diet and given the same diet training and lost four to five pounds over the course of the study.

Diet + exercise + no hormone replacement = no weight loss
Diet + exercise + natural hormone = weight loss

Additionally, the estrogen-treated group had improvements in cholesterol, glucose tolerance, and insulin sensitivity. It is of interest that the metabolic rate did not change between the two groups, and the rate of glucose burn did not change enough to explain the difference.

Another study, published in 1997 by the Endocrine Society, evaluated various popular hormone regimens but did not have participants implement lifestyle changes. The study included four groups: placebo, horse estrogen only, horse estrogen plus synthetic progestin, and horse estrogen plus natural progesterone.

Women on estrogen only or estrogen plus progesterone gained the least weight. The results were actually not surprising, as synthetic progestin and the absence of hormones tend to induce weight gain, and progesterone aids in weight maintenance.

Another study, published in 1998 in Australia, evaluated the route of estrogen administration and weight gain or loss. The study compared oral horse estrogen to transdermal estradiol, which is the dominant, natural human estrogen.

In this crossover study, participants used both routes but at different times, with the idea being that if there was a positive outcome with one intervention and a negative outcome with the other, and the outcomes occurred in the same people with the same circumstances, then the results would be considered valid.

The study found a correlation in the use of horse estrogen and decreased lean body mass (muscle and bone), as well as increased fat mass—in other words, typical aging weight adjustments. In the topically applied, natural estrogen regimen, there was improved lean body mass and no fat gain.

In summary, no hormone replacement leads to weight gain, and in most cases that weight is fat. With horse estrogen, there was less weight gain than taking nothing. With topically applied estradiol, there tends to be no fat-mass gain. And with topical estrogen plus diet changes, there is weight loss. Unfortunately, with diet alone and no hormone replacement, it is very hard to lose weight, and weight gain is pretty much a given over time.

No hormone replacement = weight gain
Horse estrogen = less weight gain
Topically applied estradiol = no weight gain
Topical estrogen + diet changes = weight loss

Another study looked at the circulating hormone levels of women on or off of HRT. The study from the University of Alabama at Birmingham, published in *Obesity* in 2012, followed women for two years and focused on the connection of hormones and the most dangerous fat—intra-abdominal adipose tissue, also known as *visceral fat*—inside the abdominal wall. Outwardly, this tissue commonly gives men a "beer belly" and can make a woman look as if she's pregnant.

Intra-abdominal adipose tissue is an inflammatory fat that leads to diseases such as certain cancers and heart disease, and it is clearly linked to type 2 diabetes, which is also called *noninsulin dependent diabetes or adult-onset diabetes.*

The researchers were looking into the hormone changes that take place from conventional HRT using horse estrogen, taken orally. Again, horse estrogen does work for menopausal symptoms and is used more commonly than a widely available human estrogen, in part because of its huge brand-name presence. While estradiol is a healthy, human estrogen, estrone is a known problem estrogen that is found in horse estrogen and is linked to breast cancer and inflammation.

Participants in the study took either a placebo or horse estrogen plus progestin.

The hormones measured during this two-year observational study of women in menopause included estradiol, estrone, testosterone, SHBG, and cortisol. Researchers took blood to measure hormone levels, and to measure abdominal fat, they used a special type of CT scan.

The study found that blood estradiol levels correlated to less abdominal fat, and estrone correlated to more abdominal fat. It also found that oral estrogens raised SHBG and cortisol levels, and both of these were positively correlated to increased visceral belly fat.

The researchers expected that increased testosterone levels would also lead to visceral fat because of the mistaken assumption that conditions of abnormally altered hormone levels (including testosterone) were associated with conditions of obesity. But that assumption turned out to be wrong. **Normal testosterone levels were associated with less belly fat, and low testosterone levels were associated with increased visceral belly fat.**

Low testosterone= increased visceral belly fat
Testosterone replacement=fat loss and improved body mass

Looking at the testosterone connection further, a study conducted in Vienna, Austria, assessed the effect of androgen replacement on weight and body composition in postmenopausal women. Androgens, again, are a class of hormones of which testosterone is the most dominant.

The study involved two groups of menopausal women: a placebo control group and a group given an androgen cream applied to the skin. The researchers performed blood laboratory determinations as well as extensive measurements to assess weight and body-mass changes.

With no other interventions, the study found that the placebo group had no significant changes in body fat or lean mass. Meanwhile, the androgen-treated group experienced beneficial changes in fat loss, abdominal fat, and lean body mass. There were no adverse effects.

Androgens, namely testosterone, are critical hormones for healthy women. Testosterone is a dominant hormone in youth and declines with age at the same time that diseases and weight gain occur. At my practice, we prescribe testosterone for all women who are deficient. We view it as a critical hormone in menopause and aging.

• •

Judy: Bioidentical—the Only Choice

For Judy, bioidenticals were the only choice when it came to HRT. "My mother had breast cancer in her fifties, so taking synthetics was a real concern," she said.

Judy first visited Allure Medical Spa for help with her varicose veins. But when perimenopausal symptoms—tiredness, weight gain, and an overall rundown feeling—kicked in while Judy was in her late forties, she returned to Allure for help.

Initially she was prescribed testosterone and progesterone, until a six-month checkup revealed that her pregnenolone levels were also low. She also had started with testosterone in the form of sublingual drops, but she switched to pellets as soon as they were offered by Allure.

Ten years since she first went to Allure, Judy continues to receive treatment for what are now menopausal symptoms. In addition to testosterone pellet implants, she continues to take progesterone, pregnenolone, and supplements, which have resolved her low libido, stress, fatigue, brain fog, and sleep problems. "They seem to be doing the trick," she said.

Today, she has plenty of energy to deal with whatever her account executive job or family issues bring her way. After having no stamina for home, work, or working out, Judy now has the energy she needs to deal with family, her job, and her lifelong love of exercise. "It's just given me an all-around sense of well-being," she said. "Now I have the energy to deal with everything."

• •

Diabetes and Metabolic Syndrome

Diabetes is a progressive disease. In this section we are talking about Type II diabetes which is also known as Adult Onset Diabetes. Although there are some genetics involved, it is mostly caused by lifestyle choices. And unfortunately, the American diet is a huge cause of diabetes. However, age and hormones influence diabetes as well.

I will talk about how a decline in hormone production leads to increased frequency of diabetes and how maintaining more youthful hormones through supplementation can help aid the fight against obesity, metabolic syndrome, and diabetes.

The first phase in a person acquiring diabetes is the development of belly, or visceral, fat. Then comes metabolic syndrome, where insulin no longer has the desired effect of normalizing and redistributing glucose (sugar). This phase is also known as insulin resistance. Then comes diabetes, the phase in which the sugar level is elevated, leading to harmful effects on all organ systems and eventually organ failure and death.

Prior to 2016, most studies looked at whether hormone replacement could mitigate or reverse diabetes-causing weight gain that is associated with menopause. A study published in 2016 wanted to take that query a step further.

Women enrolled in the three-month study were in menopause and had adult-onset type 2 diabetes.

While there are some exceptions, type 2 is an acquired form of diabetes that follows a path. First, the individual gains weight, primarily composed of visceral belly fat, from excess sugar and simple carbohydrate consumption. The muscle cells then get exposed to too much sugar and lose their responsiveness to insulin. The fat then soaks up the insulin and sugar, whereby diabetes sets in. Although dietary changes can sometimes control diabetes onset, without those changes, diabetes is likely imminent.

In the 2016 study, one group received a placebo, and the other received oral estrogen plus a synthetic progestin. The study found that women taking estrogen had better glucose control and better insulin sensitivity. They also had better HbA1c, a marker that diabetes is under control.

Hormone replacement is not an alternative for managing lifestyle. But as I mentioned, weight gain is very common during menopause—it is the most common complaint I see, well before hot flashes and night sweats. At best, it's difficult to manage your weight without hormone replacement, and treatment with human-based hormones that resemble what you used to make on your own works best. In most cases, a woman's weight will increase without HRT.

In many cases, diabetes is the natural outcome of unchecked weight gain, but hormone replacement can reduce that risk.

Treatment with long-term, human-identical hormone replacement also reduces mortality from heart attacks by over 70 percent. Heart disease is, of course, an end game of diabetes.

There are a number of other facets to weight gain that you need to know.

Contributing Factors

There are a number of factors contributing to skyrocketing obesity and extreme obesity rates in recent years. In a 2009 article in *Critical Reviews in Food Science and Nutrition* titled "Ten Putative Contributors to the Obesity Epidemic," various experts identified several causes—including "the Big Two" (diet and exercise)—but none of the causes alone could be considered the major cause of Americans and people around the planet gaining so much weight. Here are a few potentially contributing factors:

Restaurant dining and fast food—A 2008 study found that diners typically consumed two hundred to three hundred more calories at fast-food restaurants than they would at nonrestaurant meals. The study also found that diners compensated for the extra calories by eating less at other meals or skipping some eating opportunities. The net gain was about twenty-four additional calories on fast-food days. While the findings may indicate a cofactor, they certainly don't point to the only cause for obesity rates tripling in three decades.

Physical education—Lack of physical education is blamed as a cause for childhood obesity. Three other studies critically reviewed as part of the 2008 study found that kids engage in nearly the same amount of sport play. So here again, this cannot be the major cause.

High fructose corn syrup—The American Medical Association produced a position paper that high fructose corn syrup had no disadvantage over regular table sugar, and today the overall consumption of these sugars hasn't changed collectively. While this may be partly responsible, we can assume there are other factors for tripling obesity rates in less than twenty years.

Vending machines in schools—A study published in 2014 by researchers at the University of Illinois and Harvard and Cambridge Universities evaluated the impact of "sin taxes" on soda and fast food as a way of regulating children's eating behaviors in an effort to prevent obesity. Various municipalities have regulated soft-drink sizes and vending machines in schools and have placed taxes on fast food and sugary drinks. Even today, the efforts of such legislation have been unsuccessful at reducing childhood obesity.

The study evaluated the presence or absence of vending machines in schools and looked at children's consumption of sugary drinks and fast food. The study found that children who had access to sugary drinks via a vending machine at school drank significantly less soda than kids with no access to vending machines. And more interestingly, kids with access to vending machines containing sugary drinks ate fast-food less often than kids who had no access.

It's easy to imagine why this occurs: availability creates no demand, but lack of access leads to finding alternative options. Perhaps a lack of vending machines leads to kids venturing out to fast food places, where sugary drinks are a part of the experience.

Maternal age and obesity—Children born to mothers who are over age thirty have a bit more fat on them than children born to younger mothers. There are various explanations for this factor, which may include that more mature mothers may be more affluent and have more access to food, or they may be busy at work so there is less mother–child interaction.

Sleep patterns—There is a link between less sleep and higher rates of obesity over the past forty years. Lack of sleep is associated with decreased ability for the body to handle and process sugar, increases in stress hormones, and decreases in positive hormones. While sleep deprivation is a cofactor of obesity, here again, it's not the main cause.

Endocrine disruptors and toxins—These are much-maligned (rightly so) chemicals that alter hormone signaling. You may have heard about the harmful effects of Bisphenol A (BPA), a chemical compound used in the manufacture of food-packaging plastic. While this and other chemicals didn't cause the obesity epidemic, they did likely contribute.

Medications—Drugs to treat various conditions can lead to unintended weight gain, especially mood-altering drugs or drugs for depression, anxiety, high blood pressure, allergies, upset stomach, and even diabetes. Lifestyle changes can sometimes help a person avoid taking these medications altogether.

When all the contributing factors are added up, the sum does not equal the reality. Even though these changes have occurred in our society, they do not add up to the massive increase in obesity and super obesity that occurred between 1980 and 1998.

But a new discovery may now solve the mystery.

The Microbiota Connection

As I mentioned early in the chapter, humans have one set of DNA; the human body is one organism that is host to more than a hundred trillion microorganisms with more collective DNA than the human host. A microorganism is a single-cell entity, and most microorganisms are bacteria. The human body hosts good and bad bacteria. An infection is usually a microorganism that has overgrown and killed off the normal resident or healthy bacteria. Similarly, the human body hosts good and bad germs, and bad germs don't cause harm if the good germs keep them from overgrowing.

The trillions of bacteria that live on and in our bodies are known as microbiota. The study of microbiota is fairly recent; while the link between microbiota and health issues was more or less figured out twenty years ago, only in the last decade or so have strides been made in understanding the entity. Recent advances in DNA testing have allowed us to differentiate species of bacteria on a scale never imagined before. Since then, they have been implicated and linked to autoimmune diseases such as multiple sclerosis, rheumatoid arthritis, fibromyalgia, diabetes, and muscular dystrophy as well as obesity, cancer, and many gastrointestinal diseases.

There are an enormous number of species in the hundred-trillion-plus bacteria living in the gastrointestinal tract. Most are in the colon, also called the large bowel. They comprise a significant amount of the body's fecal matter. In fact, on average, a person carries around three pounds of bacteria at any point in time.

There are numerous disease-producing bacteria in the colon that can cause infection in other areas of the body, such as a wound. But these pathogenic bacteria are outnumbered and kept in check in the colon by the abundant healthy species there.

Biodiversity refers to having a balance of good and bad bacteria along with numerous species of benign bacteria. When biodiversity is altered and dominant, "bad" bacteria grow, leading to obesity. That's a simple way of explaining that the relative ratio and the biodiversity of bacteria actually predict obesity or normal weight. High biodiversity and a higher ratio of "good" bacteria equal normal weight. Low biodiversity and a high number of "bad" bacteria equal obesity. This is an oversimplification ("bad" and "good"), as there are countless variations, but it is a simple way to look at it. Additionally, we are learning more and more about this every day.

The key here is that the *ratio can be changed*. How is this possible?

The Discovery

Antibiotics and feces—When a person takes an antibiotic for an infection, the antibiotic kills not only the infection but also bacteria that live in the colon and other noninfection-causing, normal germs. This activity can be life threatening because it leaves a germ called Clostridium difficile (C. diff) left unchecked. C. diff is a minor bacterium in a healthy person, but when competing bacteria have been killed by the antibiotic, C. diff overgrows and can become a disease known as *pseudomembranous colitis*, which is manifested by severely protracted diarrhea, dehydration, and occasionally, if not managed, death.

Powerful antibiotics can sometimes treat C. diff, but when they fail, the solution is to do a fecal transplant. It sounds gross, I know, but this treatment is still the best tool for combating what is an otherwise untreatable disease. The way the treatment works is for someone in the immediate family to donate feces that are then placed into the colon of the infected person. That donated feces is loaded with normal bacteria that compete for energy and survival with the

C. diff. Ultimately, the treatment establishes a normal bacteria count in the colon. However, that colony is the same as the person who donated their feces, so *if the donor is thin, the person treated becomes thin. And if the donor is obese, then the person treated becomes obese.* In short, if you are really sick and need a fecal transplant, then you may become the size of the donor.

• •

Mouse Poop Can Be a Good Thing

The fecal transplant was actually discovered through studies of mice. Mice inherit the germs of their mother's birth canal. Normal-weight mice are born of normal-weight mothers. Overweight mice are born of overweight mothers.

Scientists fed normal-weight mice normal chow diets. Then they overfed mice born to overweight mothers.

When the normal-size mice were given fecal transplants from the overweight mice, they became overweight, even with no change in their food.

When overweight mice were given fecal transplants of the germ-free or normal-weight mice, they became normal weight in spite of being overfed.

Basically, the scientists could shape the weight of the mice by altering the makeup of their gut bacteria via feces.

• •

So how does that happen? It has to do with the way that a body and its hundreds of trillions of bacteria respond to carbohydrates, fats, and protein.

LOW-CARB VERSUS HIGH-CARB DIETS

There's a lot of misinformation out there about these three components of a person's diet—carbohydrates, fats, and protein. While some of the products or fads marketed may actually help you lose weight in the short term, restriction of any one of the three will fail as a long-term weight-loss plan.

Many carbs (carbohydrates) are polysaccharides—*poly* means "many," *saccharides* more or less means "sugar molecules." Carbs and polysaccharides are too large and complex to be properly absorbed. So the digestive track tries to break them down into oligosaccharides—*oligo* means "a few." But oligosaccharides are also too large and complex to be absorbed.

So the body then tries to break them down into monosaccharides—*mono* means "one." Monosaccharides can be digested.

But wait, there's more. Fiber and resistant starches are able to bypass the usual poly ➔ oligo ➔ mono processing system of our body. These carbs (saccharides) make it to the large bowel (the colon), where fecal bacteria break them into short-chain fatty acids (SCFAs), which are easier to absorb. Depending on the makeup of the gut microbiota, the fibers and undigested food may be turned into harmful toxins—exotoxins, immunotoxins, and endotoxins—when there is a lack of biodiversity or, in the case of beneficial high biodiversity, into anti-inflammatory SCFA.

So some carbs are absorbed as carbs while others are absorbed as fatty acids that liberate either toxins or anti-inflammatory molecules.

That's a little about carbs, and I'll talk about fats and proteins a little later in the chapter.

The Human Microbiome

Again, the gastrointestinal tract—particularly the colon—is colonized with bacteria. These bacteria operate in a symbiotic fashion. In other words, we need them, and they definitely need us.

The bacteria are responsible for up to 30 percent of the nutrients that we absorb from food. They also have a role in hormone production, which I'll discuss later in the chapter.

To better understand absorption, try this: Hold a thin wafer of bread in your mouth. As it dissolves, your oral mucosa (the pink tissue in your mouth) absorbs it. The bread is highly processed to allow easy digestion though the mouth and basically breaks down into sugar, which the body either burns off or stores.

Next, hold a white kidney bean in your mouth. Not only does the thickness of the bean's wall prevent your saliva from breaking it down, but even when it is exposed to stomach acid and small intestines attempt to absorb it, it passes right through to the colon. This is partly because of the nature of the fiber coating, but the bean also has an amylase inhibitor. Amylase is an enzyme in the mouth and gastrointestinal tract that helps digest carbohydrates. Once the bean makes it to the large bowel, your bacteria go to work breaking it down into SCFAs that are readily absorbed.

In the process of the colonic bacterial food breakdown, the germs allow for the absorption of various nutrients and beneficial fatty acids, and based on the types of dominant bacteria, can also help absorb harmful cytotoxins, genotoxins, and immunotoxins. So again, good bacteria give us nutrients and anti-inflammatory compounds, and bad bacteria give us toxins.

Add to that the fact that the good bacteria are relatively hungry and inefficient, so they burn a lot of the calories that you eat. These are flushed away when you go to the bathroom, and they must be replaced. Again, more calories are burned by the bacteria's reproduction, so if the good bacteria are dominant in the colon, the person will tend to be lean. Bad bacteria, on the other hand, are not particularly hungry, and therefore they pass most of the calories that a person consumes on to the body. If the colon is dominated by bad bacteria, the person will tend toward obesity.

Bowel with good bacteria = leanness, anti-inflammatory, free fatty acids
Bowel with bad bacteria = obesity and toxins

Microbiota and Diabetes

Now that you know more about the causative connection between gut microbiota and obesity (or leanness), let's discuss microbiota and diabetes.

First, a little background on diabetes. There are two major types of diabetes. The most common is type 2, which is known as *adult onset* and is associated with obesity. With type 2, as I discussed earlier, there is resistance to insulin and blood sugars rise dangerously. There is a genetic component to type 2 diabetes, but for the most part, type 2 diabetes is considered to be preventable by maintaining a healthy weight.

The other type of diabetes is type 1, which typically arises in childhood. Type 1 diabetes is the inability to make insulin, which also causes blood sugar to rise dangerously.

Type 1 diabetes is a complex, serious illness. It is an autoimmune disease, meaning that the body's immune system attacks itself. In this case, the insulin-secreting islet cells of the pancreas are the victims. The immune system is supposed to watch for germs and other threats. In the case of autoimmune disease, the same immune system is mistakenly attacking part of the body that is perfectly normal—in this case, parts of the pancreas.

Animal studies in mice and rats have shown a clear pattern of an unhealthy biodiversity of microbiota and patterns of certain bacteria as being present in the gut of animals that were likely to develop diabetes. In other words, the altered bacteria could predict the development of diabetes; the diabetes did not cause the alteration.

Human and animal studies have shown the propensity for autoimmune response that occurs when certain people consume gluten or cow's milk. This same pattern has been observed in patients with type 1 diabetes.

In animal studies, the development of type 1 diabetes was controlled—turned on or off—by adding or subtracting gluten or cow's milk. In the cow's milk, the protein was the likely autoimmune-causing component.

In human studies, children with type 1 diabetes who were put on a gluten-free diet became healthier, had more sensitivity to insulin, and saw improvement in their HbA1c, which is the marker of stable diabetes.

Studies have also shown that children with a high genetic risk of type 1 diabetes had altered gut flora that was less diverse and was similar to the pattern seen in animals and that children who actually developed type 1 diabetes had unhealthy patterns of fecal flora.

The research is very new and only gives a glimpse as to the cause of the devastating autoimmune disorder that is diabetes.

Inflammatory Bowel Disease— The Gut Flora Connection

A number of other autoimmune diseases have patterns of symbiosis similar to inflammatory bowel disease, so let's look at its connection to gut flora.

Two principal types of gut disease include ulcerative colitis, which typically involves only the large bowel, and Crohn's disease, which can occur in a patchy fashion throughout the bowel. These are both different from irritable bowel syndrome, which is not inflammatory.

The cause of inflammatory bowel disease appears to be linked to genetic components along with an abnormal immune response toward the bacteria in the gut.

Inflammatory bowel disease is manifested by altered permeability of the intestines. Normally, the intestines regulate fluid and nutrient flow from the gut to the body, but in the inflammatory state, where the immune system is attacking the microbiota, this permeability is altered. People with inflammatory bowel disease suffer from abdominal distress, diarrhea, and dehydration and can even die from it. My mother had ulcerative colitis and almost died at age twenty-nine from a severe form of it known as *toxic megacolon*, where her colon almost blew up. Her entire large bowel was removed through emergency surgery, and she has lived a happy, successful life with a colostomy bag ever since. She even dedicated her life to helping other people who suffered from the same condition.

A typical, American, high-fat, and high-sugar diet is a risk factor not only for inflammatory and toxin-producing bacteria but also for the development of inflammatory bowel disease.

Promising therapy is aimed at resorting optimal bacteria, altering the diet from a typical American diet to a cleaner diet, and the use of probiotics. I'll talk about diet later in the chapter.

The Human Microbiome and Cancer

Extensive scientific evidence has unequivocally linked the American, or Western, diet to many cancers.

One comprehensive look at the data was published in 2006 in *The China Study: The Most Comprehensive Study of Nutrition Ever Conducted and the Startling Implications for Diet, Weight Loss, and Long-Term Health*, by T. Colin Campbell and Thomas M. Campbell. This book looked at the extensive data collected by the emperor of China decades ago, combined with a revisit in this century of the same data and patterns. The data reveals that certain cancers were extremely low in cultures that had virtually no access to animal protein, whereas cultures with access to an American diet tended to have Western diseases, including premature heart disease and colon, breast, and prostate cancer. The book somewhat predates the link to microbiota as the "why" for the diseases.

In 2015, the World Health Organization also identified processed meats such as hot dogs, ham, bacon, sausage, and some deli meats as definitive carcinogens and listed red meats as probable carcinogens.

Casein, one of the proteins found in milk, has also been shown in numerous studies to promote the growth of cancer.

Another interesting article, "The Microbiome and Cancer," published in 2013 in the *National Reviews Cancer*, evaluated the evidence relating the human microbiome and cancer and sought to further the understanding why there is such a strong link. The research was designed to find out why certain foods can give us cancer, and the data appears to show that gut microbiome plays a role.

Other studies and scientific review papers have focused on specific cancers. A 2014 article in the *World Journal of Oncology* looked at the effect of diet patterns on the microbiota and how they relate to the development of breast cancer. The study noted how the consumption of certain foods altered the microbiota and protected against breast cancer, as well as how consumption of other foods negatively impacted the microbiota and led to increased rates of breast cancer.

Other studies have shown a connection between the gut microbiota and the risk of colorectal cancer, as well as a link between the microbiota and likelihood of survival after successful treatment of the cancer.

The Hormone Connection

To help you get a better understanding of the interplay between the gut microbiome, obesity, and sexual hormones, let's return to studies on mice.

Before talking about the connection between male and female mice in this subject, let me first talk about male mice and the relationship of gastrointestinal bacteria and testosterone. A look at male hormones was the first step in the discovery of the link between microbiota, hormones, and health.

In males, testosterone is made in the testicles through what are called Leydig cells. With age, these cells become less healthy, which leads to declining androgen levels, a condition known as "male menopause" or "andropause." Although not as abrupt as menopause, there is a relationship between lowering testosterone levels in men and the onset of obesity, decreased sexual desire and performance, diabetes, heart disease, depression, loss of mental sharpness, and various other undesirable conditions associated with aging.

In an interesting study supported by the NIH and carried out at Harvard, the Massachusetts Institute of Technology, and other institutes of higher learning, the use of probiotics was studied in mice for its potential health benefits.

Probiotics are bacteria that are beneficial to the host organism. they are commonly sold at any drug store, mostly in a pill form. They are used to restore healthy bacteria after conditions in the gut impair the existing bacteria.

Researchers in this study noticed that the mice given probiotics looked younger and had more "luxuriant hair." These changes were in comparison to the siblings of the mice, which were given a placebo and had normal age-related changes such as thinning hair, an aged look, and weight gain when fed high-calorie diets.

The study also found that the placebo mice gained weight when put on the higher-calorie diet, whereas the probiotic mice were resistant to obesity. They also evaluated the effect of the probiotic (and the placebo) on serum testosterone levels and found a profound correlation. The mice eating the probiotics had substantially higher testosterone levels than those given placebos.

The study found that the beneficial effect of the probiotic supplementation acted by preventing the inflammation that normally occurs when calories are digested. The higher bacteria diversity brought on by the addition of probiotics prevented testicular shrinkage, preserved testosterone levels, and protected against obesity.

Another study published around the same time looked at male mice. Instead of supplementing with probiotics, researchers evaluated germ-free versus normal mice. The study had pretty similar findings: mice without bacteria (germ-free mice) had lower testosterone levels than mice with microbiota and also exhibited failure of the testicles to fully form. This finding demonstrated that the gut bacteria are influential in the creation of sex hormones.

Although males and females are different, this set the stage for the understanding that hormones and our gut bacteria were crucially linked. The fact that bacteria had a substantial impact on the testosterone in male mice led researchers to investigate the female hormone connection to microbiota.

In 2015, researchers from Colorado State University wanted to find out more about the relationship between declining estrogen levels in women, loss of gut diversity, and the increasing risks of obesity, diabetes, and cardiac disease.

The researchers divided female rats into two groups. One group had their ovaries removed; the other had a sham surgery where they were opened up but had nothing removed. This was done to avoid questions as to whether it's the act of an abdominal procedure or the actual removal of an organ that accounts for a difference between groups. There were also two different populations of rats studied: ones that were bred to run on a wheel in their cage and others that had no interest in such an activity. The two groups were fed the same diet.

The study found that the rats with their ovaries removed gained weight. Not surprisingly, the rats with the running tendency gained less than the inactive rats. The sham surgery rats experienced no weight changes.

As for the microbiota, there was a correlation to an unfavorable trend after the ovaries were removed, and the rats that were more inclined to exercise saw less change. Here again is a link between microbiota—the third cause of obesity—and alterations in hormone levels.

Another study, conducted around the same time on rats in the Midwest, looked at more or less the same conditions. When the animals had their ovaries removed and hence experienced a precipitous drop in their hormones, the gut microbiota changed to an unfavorable status. Exercise could reduce the intensity of the change, but there was still an unfavorable change.

In another study on rats that included three groups—two groups with their ovaries removed and a third group with ovaries intact—researchers looked specifically at bone mass loss, a typical outcome of ovarian removal or failure. The rats were fed either placebo or probiotics; placebo-fed rats with ovaries removed had typical bone loss, which was averted when the animals were fed probiotics.

So it is not just the abrupt loss of estrogen that leads to bone failure: it is the interaction of the gut microbiota and estrogen that ultimately decides the fate. While weight gain is a significant concern for women entering or in menopause, gut microbiota (the third cause of obesity) is also altered by a drop in youthful sexual hormones.

Gut microbiota is instrumental in the genesis and composition of various hormones. Again, estrogen is synthesized from other hormones, notably androgens including testosterone. Many—perhaps all—organ systems are capable of synthesizing estrogen. Some organs such as fat cells may tend to make more undesirable estrogens, while others make healthier estrogens.

Estrogens in the body are continuously excreted in the urine or by the liver in the form of bile. Bile wanders through the entire digestive track, and bile estrogen passes to the intestines, where it is fair game for the microbiota. There, bacteria can alter the type of estrogen that is present, the altered estrogen reabsorbs into the body, and the body then uses the estrogen in its altered form. Eventually, the altered estrogens are permanently excreted in the urine.

What one study found was that women with a high biodiversity of microbiota tended to have healthy estrogens. Women with a low biodiversity tended toward harmful estrogen metabolites.

A healthy gut helps maintain healthy estrogens in postmenopausal women. Gut microbiota, as studies have shown, is a lynchpin to overall health, not just to maintaining a healthy weight.

Better Gut Microbiota

The amazing discovery of the interplay between our microbiota and health is very recent, and more studies are coming out at an amazing pace from numerous universities. But the subject itself is very new, and before solutions are identified and discovered, there must necessarily be more research into why and how the interplay occurs in the first place. In summarizing where we are today, I also want to share with you the direction we're headed with this exciting new discovery. As I write this book, there is no magic bullet; there is no antibiotic, probiotic, or slam-dunk food or diet that can rapidly alter your gut microbiota into a perfectly healthy one. However, there is evidence that making consistent minor changes can have a positive impact on your own gut microbiota, and hence your weight and overall health.

• •

Our Own Research Project

Because we're at the threshold of such an exciting discovery, we've decided to conduct our own research project at my practice.

I recently had a dinner meeting with a doctoral researcher from the University of Michigan microbiome department. During our chat, we discussed the broad difference in our patients. His are mice, whose genetics, environment, food, and level of activity are chosen by design. My patients, of course, have free will—their genetics are set, and they make their own choices about environment, food, and level of activity.

That choice is what our in-office research boils down to. Science has shown us that our microbiota is affected not only by what we eat, our hormone levels, and other exposures but also by our community and family. In other words, it seems to be contagious—the microbiota in your body can take on the resemblance of those you spend time with.

For some time, we have used our local premium grocery store, Vince and Joe's, as a private chef to make healthy meals for our staff, which they can choose whether or not to eat. We have a smoothie machine and a fridge full of greens on site, and we'll pay the majority of membership dues for anyone in our office who wants to join the premium gyms in our areas (Lifetime Fitness). About half of our staff takes advantage of these perks.

Recently we added three new perks, which most of our staff are adding to their intake: one tablespoon daily of: spinach thylakoids, which are basically freeze-dried spinach membranes; galacto-oligosaccharide, which is a soluble, nondigestible fiber designed to help grow "good" bacteria; and a selected series of probiotics. I'll talk about how these work a bit later.

The goal is to see if over the long term, in a work setting, we can create a healthier workforce. About 20 percent of our staff is participating by choice. Many staff members have their families participate as well, but we are not tracking them.

In the short term, we found that people participating in our "experiment" are losing about one pound per month. Participants have noticed less hunger and improved mood. One person even retested her thyroid panel recently and found that she is now completely free of her Hashimoto's antibodies. Initially, many people had mild gastric distress, which is related to the shifting of the microbiota—hopefully to a healthier one. But that distress goes away. Long term, we are going to measure the effect of deliberately attempting to alter our practice's microbiota to a collectively healthy one.

• •

Synbiotics—Probiotics and Prebiotics

Synbiotics refers to combinations of probiotics and prebiotics.

As I mentioned earlier, probiotics are beneficial bacteria that you consume. They are created in a lab and made to be ingested. Numerous studies have shown beneficial effects of taking probiotics on certain disease states. The idea is that a person eats the bacteria, the bacteria hopefully take hold and grow, and then they eventually alter the composition of the person's microbiota.

Prebiotics are chemical compounds in foods that influence the microbiota.

Because I am personally biased toward prebiotics—I prefer to think of "food as medicine"—we routinely counsel patients on proper nutrition. We have handouts, videos, and educational tools for patients so they can understand what foods are proven to be the most healthy and nutrient dense.

Probiotics research—In 2016, a large meta-analysis paper was published by the University of Granada, Spain. A meta-analysis is a thorough review of all the available, relevant, peer-reviewed, and consistent studies. The study was to identify the evidence, or lack thereof, for the use of probiotics on the treatment of obesity, insulin resistance, type 2 diabetes, and obesity-related liver disease—conditions that typically occur after the onset of menopause.

The studies analyzed administered about ten billion bacteria per dose daily, which is far more than is in supplemented yogurt or most available probiotic capsules. The human microbiome contains many strains and substrains of bacteria. The strains in most probiotics are *Lactobacillus*, which doesn't correlate well to the presence or absence of obesity. But *Lactobacillus* is widely available, is found in many healthy foods, and is present in the gastrointestinal tract. There are also substrains of *Lactobacillus*. In fact, it is so common that a probiotic label may read simply: "*L. salivarius*" or "*L. acidophilus*" where the "L" stands for "*Lactobacillus*."

In the meta-analysis, it was discovered that some of the common *Lactobacillus* used in various studies on obese children and obese postmenopausal women had no effect. However, other probiotics had favorable effects on obesity, insulin resistance, and type 2 diabetes. For probiotics to have an effect on weight loss, there must be a high number of bacteria, and they must be taken for greater than eight weeks. Some strains seem to work better than others, and we recommend using several strains.

In a 2010 study, they followed subjects who consumed fifty billion colony-forming units (CFUs) of the bacteria L. gasseri. A CFU is the measurement of the dosage with probiotics, and CFUs are able to divide and replicate themselves.

The subjects in the study, who consumed the L. gasseri daily for twelve weeks, saw a reduction in body mass index (BMI), specifically a reduction in harmful visceral (belly) fat.

Another study of more than two hundred people evaluated L. gasseri at a higher dose of one hundred billion CFU daily for twelve weeks. The study participants saw a decrease of the same parameters: lower BMI (meaning a drop in obesity) and a reduction in belly fat.

Two other studies looked at another probiotic, L. plantarum. In one study, the subjects were given 150 billion CFU a day and saw a favorable drop in both BMI and blood pressure. Participants in the other study took ninety billion CFU a day and saw no effect. This points to not only the strain of probiotic but also the number consumed daily as influencing factors.

Other studies used a variety of probiotics in combination, and all had subtle but favorable effects on the attributes being studied. These studies were good evidence for microbiota biodiversity being the common link. Numerous other studies have shown favorable improvements on cardiac lipids such as LDL, HDL, and total cholesterol. Additionally, probiotics have shown improved glucose and insulin interaction.

Prebiotics research—Prebiotics are nondigestible fibers found in foods. Prebiotics pass through the digestive tract and are eventually consumed by gut microbiota. Healthy prebiotics breed a healthy microbiota. Probiotics are bacteria; prebiotics are foods that good bacteria want to digest in order to reproduce.

There are commercially available prebiotics in powder or pill form. But most of the research has been done on the effect of actual foods—not supplements—on the gut microbiota.

Probiotics plus prebiotics—When prebiotics are added to probiotics, the results are more profound.

In studies of obese children, probiotics alone did nothing for management of obesity. But when probiotics were combined with prebiotics, two studies showed decreases in BMI, waist circumference, and other measurements of obesity.

Studies of adults produced the same results, netting fairly consistent improvements in aspects of obesity. When evaluating insulin resistance, probiotics tended to work, but not consistently. However, prebiotics together with probiotics improved fasting blood sugar and insulin resistance significantly.

For type 2 diabetes, probiotics trended toward improved blood glucose and insulin, whereas probiotics together with prebiotics produced more consistent improvements in similar areas.

At the writing of this book, probiotics continue to be an interesting area of research but one where there is still much to be understood: What is the best dose? What strain or substrain is best? Does taking a variety of strains offer a benefit? Does *Lactobacillus* offer the best benefits? Or do we need more Bifidobacterium, or another, yet unknown favorable bacteria?

For the prebiotics, we recommend a green smoothie at least once daily, which you blend with the highest nutritionally dense foods. Do not add processed food such as protein powder.

As for probiotics, look for a high count (over fifty billion) and a variety of strains of *Lactobacillus* and *Bifidobacterium*.

If you do not have a green smoothie, you can use a prebiotic powder. Our office is using galacto-oligosaccharide (one teaspoon a day). When you start a prebiotic, there can be gastric distress, as your favorable bacteria may be dominated by unfavorable bacteria. Unfavorable bacteria will convert the prebiotic into gas and other substances. The favorable bacteria will convert the prebiotic into healthy, free fatty acids. This is a simplification but is basically what happens. To avoid gastric distress when taking prebiotics, begin by taking probiotic capsules for two weeks, and then start the prebiotic in tiny doses and increase as tolerated.

For our patients seeking weight loss, we use the same system that we are using in our long-term experiment with office staff. We recommend making a vegetable smoothie every day; the list of ingredients is in the following table.

We recommend the spinach thylakoids and galacto-oligosaccharide (or other prebiotic fiber), and we use different probiotic formulas. I am still working on the best probiotic.

To put this in perspective, let me share with you a story about weight loss not associated with menopause.

At my practice, we offer patients a gastric balloon procedure that involves using a scope to insert a balloon into the stomach. When inflated, the balloon is approximately the size and shape of a grapefruit. The procedure is designed to help people who have had no success with diet and exercise programs lose weight. It's for people who have repeatedly failed at their efforts to lose weight but who are not so obese that they would qualify for weight-loss surgery.

Once the balloon is inserted, patients are supposed to take the three supplements—spinach thylakoids, galacto-oligosaccharide (or other prebiotic fiber), and a probiotic—and return to the office weekly to report on any changes to their lifestyle.

At six months, the balloon is extracted. Tanya, our nurse, measures the results of our patients who have the procedure done. Patients who were not compliant—meaning they came in the office for accountability less than eight times in six months—lost an average of twelve pounds. Patients who were compliant to some degree lost an average of thirty-six pounds. And those who were compliant consistently lost far more weight.

The moral of the story is that tools can help, but there is no alternative to commitment.

Other Lifestyle Interventions

While prebiotics and probiotics will likely yield some benefit, gut flora can also be controlled by dietary choices. Some are pretty obvious, and some are fairly surprising. Here are some of the current popular diet strategies tried by women in menopause suffering from weight gain:

Low-calorie diets—There are different terms for the numerous low-calorie diets that are trending as I write this book. One of the more prominent is the human chorionic gonadotropin (hCG) diet, which claims to be able to reset the body's metabolism so the dieter can lose up to one pound a day without feeling hungry or getting weak. For eight weeks, a person attempting this diet limits herself to five hundred calories per day while taking hCG treatments, which are administered as a shot, drops, pellets, or spray.

Studies showed that people certainly lost weight on this diet, but the hCG had no impact and is exactly the same as a placebo.

Whatever forms they take or names they goes by, five-hundred-calorie diets have popped up every now than since the 1950s. Commonly, these diets undergo multiple studies that show they have no benefit over the placebo used in the research, yet they continue to be popular every time they rear their heads.

Many of these diets are not approved by the FDA—in fact, the hCG diet has earned itself a special black-box warning telling physicians not to prescribe it for weight loss because it is a ruse.

And even though super-low-calorie diets tend to work, it's the very low consumption of calories that causes people to lose weight—typically not the supplement used. Unfortunately, because these diets don't typically lead to healthy habits, the weight is usually put back on. A number of my patients have had short-term success with these diets but no success in the long term. We do not recommend them.

Periodic fasting—These diets involve fasting or only having very low-calorie meals one to two days a week with normal but healthy food intake on the remaining days. These diets are likely to have a beneficial effect on the gut microbiota and can help with weight loss. They are less likely (compared to longer-term, very low-calorie diets) to lower your metabolism. I have tried this, and so have a few of my friends who are constantly experimenting with healthy lifestyles. It is very difficult. The alternate-day fasting leads to substantial hunger.

Meal-replacement diets—These diets essentially involve consuming more protein powder and skipping meals. Meal-replacement diets can certainly help a woman lose weight, especially if she is obese. But as with severely calorie-restrictive diets, in the long-term, these diets are doomed to fail. One of the biggest problems with meal-replacement diets is that they change the gut microbiota in a negative way. Typically, weight management after the diet is far more difficult because the microbiota has been altered to have less biodiversity. We do not endorse these diets.

Extremely low-fat diets—These diets were very popular in the 1980s and ultimately led to a cultural change where now store shelves are lined with "low-fat" junk food such as cookies, cakes, and ice cream. Obviously, the ploy did not work. Why? Because fats were substituted with simple carbohydrates, which we now know have a negative effect on gut microbiota, leading to weight gain. We do not recommend these diets.

High-protein diets—Today, high-protein diets are dominant in our culture. But do these high-protein diets work in the long term?

Certainly, if a significantly overweight woman cuts down on carbohydrates and starts eating more protein, she will initially lose weight. However, while protein—especially animal protein— is easily digested in the stomach and upper gastrointestinal tract, it lacks indigestible compounds, which are absolutely necessary for healthy gut microbiota to exist. When in menopause, a woman tends to develop unhealthy gut microbiota, so it's a key time to consume foods that promote healthy digestive microbiota. That's why high-protein diets work at first but fail in the long term, as the weight gently returns.

A 2007 study evaluated the addition of protein to the diets of postmenopausal women. Researchers gave the study participants twenty grams of soy protein or a "placebo" of casein, a form of milk protein. Casein is a slow protein that was generally assumed to lead to weight loss. And because it is so low in sugar and is a pure protein, it was assumed to be healthy and not to cause weight gain, which therefore qualified it to be a placebo. It's interesting to note that casein is the main ingredient in Greek yogurt, which is touted as a healthy weight-loss substitute to normal food.

In the study, the women were given the casein, which was considered to be a placebo, or an equal amount of soy protein. The researchers were trying to show that soy protein resulted in weight loss versus casein, which should be neutral on the weight.

At the end of three months, the woman eating casein gained five times more belly fat than the woman eating soy protein. But regardless of whether they were taking soy protein or casein protein, all of the women in the study gained fat.

Now, it's known from prior studies that casein leads to undesirable gut microbiota. In a 2007 study, researchers went with the popular belief that casein is neutral on fat or is even a health food that can be compared to soy protein for weight loss.

The bottom line is that, in spite of popular belief, protein added to the diet will not lead to long-term weight loss. There is certainly evidence, however, that adding protein to your diet can result in weight gain and is commonly used by athletes trying to gain muscle mass after intense exercise. And while there are exceptions to the rule, adding protein is not a weight-loss solution for middle-aged women. It just doesn't happen.

Also note that Greek yogurt and regular yogurt are not the same. Regular yogurt has been shown to be uniquely associated with long-term weight maintenance. Greek yogurt entered the scene as an alternative to regular yogurt with less fat and sugar, and we do not recommend it.

Another study published in 2012 sought to determine how different soy milks versus cow's milk would affect the gut microbiota in overweight and obese individuals. The study found that the cow's milk had a negative influence on the gut microbiota and led to weight gain within a short period of time. The soy milk had a favorable change in the gut microbiota, favoring bacteria that were more likely to lead to weight loss.

High-protein diets can certainly cause weight loss in some over-weight people simply because adding protein can bring more balance to a typical American diet loaded with fat and carbohydrates. However, diets high in animal protein are inflammatory and will ultimately alter the gut microbiota, leading to weight gain. Because they substantially alter the gut microbiota, they also increase the risk of inflammatory bowel disease, other autoimmune diseases, and colorectal cancer. While there is a lot of excitement about high-protein diets, I do not recommend these for any period of time.

The addition of prebiotics and high amounts of fiber can counter-teract the gut microbiota change, but in general, high-protein diets should only be used for short-term management of obesity when other methods have failed. Once the individual has experienced success with the high-protein diet, then she should switch to a more normal, healthy diet.

The Mediterranean diet is a healthy dietary option for maintaining weight. The diet includes a higher intake of nuts, vegetables, fruits, olive oil, and fibers along with a limited intake of fish and poultry. Red meats and dairy are not consumed much in the Mediterranean diet, and conservative intake of alcohol such as red wine may be included.

The Mediterranean diet has been clearly associated with weight maintenance or weight loss. It is a very anti-inflammatory diet and stimulates production of favorable gut bacteria. Considering its parameters, it makes sense that the diet would work because it limits inflammatory animal protein but includes plenty of plant protein, which is not as digestible in the human gut but is perfectly digestible by the gut microbiota. This favors the development of a diverse species of beneficial bacteria.

As this type of diet is the most solidly proven, safe, and healthy and has the best potential for long-term compliance, we recommend it to our patients.

The QR code directs you to Dr. Mok's "Nutrition 101" video to learn more about the power of healthy foods.

As part of our treatment for patients seeing us for menopause issues, we evaluate their diet and make recommendations to help them achieve optimum health. Those recommendations include a diet that is plant-based, high in anti-inflammatory foods (like the Mediterranean diet), and limiting of meats, particularly red meat. We also recommend one or two green smoothies per day, as this is a way to get a lot of green vegetables in an easy-to-manage fashion.

The Critical Role of Fiber

It is critical for women entering menopause to maintain a healthy weight, and prebiotics and fiber play key roles in that effort. As an American society we are dependent on refined grains, starches, and animal fat and protein for the majority of our calorie intake. More than two-thirds of American adults cannot maintain a normal weight on such a diet. In menopause, that statistic is even higher, signaling a critical need to make some changes.

There are two basic classifications of fiber: *soluble* and *insoluble*.

Soluble fiber more or less dissolves in water. Examples of foods containing soluble fiber are beans, peas, oats, nuts, flax seed, fruits, and many vegetables. Insoluble fibers can be found in vegetables, particularly dark, leafy greens, green beans, bell peppers, and onions. Insoluble fibers are also found in whole wheats and whole grains.

Many plant-based foods have both soluble and insoluble fibers. Animal-based foods have none. The fiber in food does not get broken down by the human system; it either passes through the bowel and becomes fecal matter or is broken down by colon bacteria. Fibers that become fecal matter are bulk-forming fibers, which reduce constipation, remove toxins, and maintain healthy intestinal pH (a measure of fluid acidity). These fibers help lower the risk of colon cancer. Fibers that are broken down by colon bacteria are fermented, becoming "fermentable fiber," which seems to be a key ingredient in growing beneficial, healthy, anti-inflammatory bacteria in the gut.

Two well-studied soluble fermentable fibers are inulin (not insulin) and oligofructose. There are plenty of other beneficial fibers, but these two have been studied the most and appear to be "super compounds." Earlier I talked about the prebiotic that we use: galacto-oligosaccharide. It is less researched and used in America, but it is common in Asia and is gaining popularity. It is easier to consume as a supplement than inulin and oligofructose. Inulin comes from chicory root and dandelion stems, and I eat them (the roots and stems) in my vegetable smoothie. But if I use inulin powder, it leads to some gastric distress. Galacto-oligosaccharide is from legumes and doesn't lead to gastric distress in most people; in fact, it is used as an additive to babies' milk to improve bowel function.

Prebiotics are soluble fermentable fibers, and they travel through your digestive tract until they encounter bacteria, which ferment them. Prebiotics are generally from the plant kingdom.

Many manufacturers are starting to create soluble fermentable fibers in powder form, making them easy to add to the diet. However, rarely are these powdered forms of fiber truly beneficial. It's better just to eat vegetables, fruits, and legumes. A diet rich in vegetables, fruits, and legumes offers the benefits of not only fermentable soluble fibers but also of phytochemicals, which bind to cell membranes and can prevent adhesion by pathogens. While I don't recommend avoiding meat altogether, the evidence is pretty clear that there are merits to having a much higher percentage of your diet's calories from plants than from animals.

The value of fiber in a high-fat diet cannot be overstated, as was proven in a 2015 study in which mice were fed either normal diets or high-fat diets. The mice were also given soluble fermentable fiber (inulin) or insoluble fiber.

In the mice that were fed normal diets, neither the soluble nor insoluble fiber group gained fat. The mice fed high-fat diets and given soluble fiber maintained a normal weight, while those given insoluble fiber became obese. Their gut microbiota also changed:

the insoluble fiber was not effective enough to block the inevitable change. Meanwhile, the mice on soluble fiber had a diversity of bacteria known to promote normal weight, which persisted in spite of a high-fat diet that bred bad germs. For a reminder, soluble fiber is the prebiotic that is digested by bacteria and found in vegetables, while insoluble fiber is found more in grains and is more commonly thought of when we say "fiber."

Another study through the University of Pennsylvania sought to determine if the differences seen globally in gut microbiota were due to environmental pressures-(i.e., location) or due to diet alone. Certain areas of the globe have high rates of obesity, and others have low rates, but researchers wanted to know if the American diet is entirely to blame for the increase in obesity worldwide.

The societies that have the lowest rates of cardiovascular diseases; diabetes; colon, prostate and breast cancer; inflammatory disease; and autoimmune disease typically eat plant-based foods as their main source of calories. Societies or global regions with high rates of the same diseases typically have high levels of animal protein consumption and generally have more fats, refined and processed foods, and sugar.

The study evaluated the gut microbiota of vegans versus a typical American diet. Vegans are people who eat a total plant-based diet with no milk, cheese, or fish. The researchers collected data from people in similar geographic areas and analyzed their fecal microbiota. The results of the study were that geographic area had nothing to do with gut microbiota, indicating that gut microbiota is entirely linked to diet.

Low-Calorie Sweeteners

Many people attempt to cut down on sugar consumption by using low-calorie sweeteners. Unfortunately, there is at least a correlation between consumption of low-calorie sweeteners—particularly in beverages—and obesity. In other words, people who are obese are much more likely to drink beverages with low-calorie sweeteners.

For a very long time, the assumption was that low-calorie sweeteners stimulated sugar cravings, thereby causing a person to consume more. But now, we know that the composition of gut microbiota determines resistance to obesity and anti-inflammatory conditions and whether a person is more prone to diseases such as glucose intolerance, diabetes, obesity, hypertension, heart disease, and inflammatory processes.

Still, researchers for the past thirty years have evaluated the response of gut microbiota to no-calorie or low-calorie artificial sweeteners. Those studies have found that artificial sweeteners do stimulate snacking by increasing cravings, but it's the negative effect on gut microbiota that tends to create the bacteria that lead to obesity, inflammation, diabetes, and disease.

Animal studies have shown that it takes a fair amount of artificial sweetener to lead to the altered gut microbiota, and human studies have shown a pretty clear link between artificial sweeteners and diseases characterized by altered gut microbiota.

There's no definitive evidence as of yet, but I recommend against using artificial sweeteners except in moderation—not that I'm promoting sugary drinks, because both are deleterious to weight and health over time.

Eating "American" VS Eating Green

If someone wants to eat like a "typical American," she will likely begin to look like one—which unfortunately means overweight or obese. The facts don't lie: two-thirds of adult Americans are overweight or obese, and there has been a dramatic shift toward that status since the 1980s.

A study of rodents looked at exposure to what was referred to as a "cafeteria diet" to determine the frequency at which the rodents would develop altered gut microbiota and gain weight when eating cafeteria-type foods, such as fried foods. The two rodent groups were fed normal chow, or the cafeteria diet. It took as few as three exposures per week to the cafeteria-style diet to develop negatively altered gut microbiota.

As I mentioned earlier, I view food as medicine. And as the studies show, it's indisputable that increasing the plant-based content of a diet will protect an individual from weight gain and other diseases associated with inflammation.

Green plants, especially, are the diet and health savior. They are abundant, readily available, and carry various types of fibers. However, green plants can be a difficult-to-acquire taste for some people. That's why I often recommend blending them into a "green shake" to break down the cell walls and make them easier to digest.

Proof of the value of a green shake can be seen in a 2014 study conducted in Sweden. The study was composed of two groups of middle-aged women who were put on the same, relatively healthy diet for twelve weeks. One of the groups began each day with a green protein drink made of five grams of dark green vegetables, a few other vegetables, and water.

After twelve weeks, the women in the control group who drank no morning green drink supplement lost around seven pounds. But the women who added in a small amount of green plant drink before breakfast had lost more than ten pounds in the same time frame. Additionally, women who drank the morning green drink had fewer cravings, for instance, for chocolate. They also felt more comfortable with what they ate. They lost more weight, and it was easier!

Further studies sought to find out why adding green plants to the diet suppressed "hedonistic hunger"—in other words, hunger or cravings even when a person should not really be hungry.

The QR code directs you to a video on "How to Make a Smoothie." Learn how to make a delicious and nutritious green drink.

One study sought to determine what compound in green leafy vegetables led to feeling fuller sooner than when eating many foods. What the study discovered was that a hormone, GLP-1, is released by certain compounds in green leafy vegetables and signals fullness.

Another study in Sweden studied thylakoids as a hunger suppressant. Thylakoids are the compounds in green plants that turn sunlight and carbon dioxide into oxygen—in other words, they are responsible for photosynthesis. In this case, the thylakoids were freeze-dried spinach leaf membranes. In the study, one group of middle-aged, overweight women was given a drink containing thylakoids, and the other group of women was given a placebo. Both groups were put on a high-fat, high-carbohydrate diet. Snacks were part of the diet, but participants could choose whether or not to eat them. The study found that women consuming the thylakoid drink ate fewer snacks (and therefore consumed fewer calories), felt less

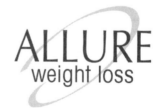

   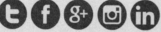

hunger, and felt full sooner. Also, interestingly, the women in the thylakoid group did not get as much pleasure from eating snacks.

A follow-up to the study found that in the women who consumed the thylakoid drink, not only was there a decrease in calorie consumption, but blood sugar levels also lowered, and the hormones associated with weight loss improved. Another follow-up study had one group using thylakoids hidden in jelly (so it couldn't be tasted) and the other group of women having just the jelly as a supplement. Both groups of women were given the same diet advice. At the end of the three-month study, both groups of women lost weight, but the women with the thylakoid supplementation lost about twice as much weight and felt it had been less difficult.

Weight gain is the most common concern I hear from women entering menopause. I have discussed how maintenance of healthy hormone levels can positively impact weight on an individual level. A bigger issue, however, is for our society as a whole to reverse the trend of obesity by being committed to changing to healthier lifestyles for every member of the family. Americans have been exposing their bodies to sugar, fat, and refined foods for so long that their guts have been infected with "fat bugs." But it doesn't have to be that way.

• •

The Winning Edge

- Weight gain typically accompanies menopause and is the cause of emotional distress as well as health risks.
- Dieting alone has little impact, if any, on menopause-induced weight gain.
- There is a clear link between levels of healthy, youthful hormones and weight maintenance. There is also a link between unhealthy hormone levels and weight gain.

- Even oral, synthetic, horse-based estrogen can slow weight gain in menopause. Changing to human-based, skin-inserted, or applied estrogen slows weight gain further. Adding estrogen to a weight-loss plan also leads to weight loss rather than gain in menopause.

- Androgens, such as testosterone, have a link to weight maintenance or weight loss.

- Not treating menopause with hormone replacement is as absurd as not treating hypothyroidism, diabetes, hypertension, or heart disease.

- Replacing hormones can help with maintaining weight and reducing the incidence of certain diseases. Diet, exercise, and maintenance of healthy hormones are a big part of understanding and managing weight gain.

- Gut microbiota can predict and cause weight gain associated with the American diet, and there is a clear link to the hormonal state of the body.

- It takes both hormone replacement and lifestyle changes to lose or maintain weight.

- Fad and high-protein diets are not the answer. A healthy diet reduces processed and cafeteria-style foods, fats and sugars, and artificial sweeteners and includes more vegetables and less meat.

- Lowering consumption of inflammatory foods and substances can help maintain healthy gut microbiota and reduce risk of diabetes, obesity, heart disease, autoimmune disease, and cancer.

· ·

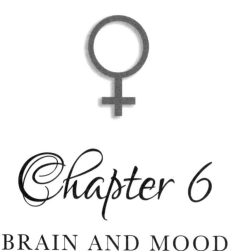

Chapter 6

BRAIN AND MOOD

Among the fears brought by the WHI trials published over a decade ago was the idea that HRT could lead to the development of dementia. Researchers found that women on CEE, or horse estrogen, plus synthetic progestin had a small but statistically significant increase in certain features related to dementia.

To reiterate, the WHI trials were conducted in a different fashion than the medicine practiced both then and now. Study participants were women who were well into menopause—generally about ten years—instead of at the onset of menopause. In the practice of medicine, hormones are started at the onset of menopause, not a decade later. Also, the women were started on HRT that consisted of horse estrogen, which was already known to have disadvantages over human estrogen. Additionally, the researchers used the totally synthetic progestin medroxyprogesterone acetate instead of the hormone progesterone, even though it was known that there were disadvantages of using a drug instead of the actual hormone it was synthesized to replace.

The WHI trials were done after years of research suggested a brain-protective nature of estrogen and other hormones. Evidence in humans and animals was contradicted in the WHI trials, and this appears to be related to the timing of the initiation of the hormone replacement.

Prior to the WHI trials, it was generally accepted that hormone replacement was protective against Alzheimer's, protected the brain from toxic attacks, and stimulated neuron formation. But ever since the results of the WHI trials were published, doubts have lingered about HRT's link to memory and aging.

So what should you believe?

HRT and Alzheimer's

To answer the question of whether HRT leads to dementia or Alzheimer's involves a meta-analysis study, which as I mentioned earlier, is a review by a team of statisticians and researchers of the published literature to answer specific questions based on all the data that can be reviewed.

In 2014, the Oxford University Press published a meta-analysis study from the Johns Hopkins Bloomberg School of Public Health, titled "Postmenopausal hormone therapy is not associated with risk of all-cause dementia and Alzheimer's disease." The intent of the article was to put to rest the controversy that started after the anomaly in the WHI study suggested that HRT use was a risk factor for developing dementia in women. There were numerous studies, of course, after the WHI trials to try to determine why the WHI women had slightly more dementia when most prior research dictated brain protection or at least a neutral effect on the brain.

The investigators in the meta-analysis used very strict criteria for the articles they were collating. For instance, the articles had to be published in peer review journals, which as I've mentioned are the gold standard for scientific and medical journals, as they tend to scrutinize papers for bias and misleading conclusions. There were other criteria as well to ensure the papers were high quality and meaningful so that clinicians could use them to make medical decisions.

The meta-analysis reviewed 2,046 articles that were related to HRT, menopause, and dementia or Alzheimer's, whittling down those to fewer than twenty that could be used to draw useful, meaningful data—and consequently, answers.

Although meta-analysis studies can be hard to read, the conclusions are important if the study is done well, which this one was.

The conclusion is that HRT for menopause, whether used for a brief period of time or the rest of a woman's life, has neither a protective nor adverse impact on either Alzheimer's disease or dementia.

For decades, women have been prescribed HRT for menopause, and in most cases receive menopause hormones that are not actual copies of human hormones. And for all of those millions of women, the studies found no added risk of dementia or Alzheimer's. *HRT was perfectly safe from a brain standpoint.* So while there was no added risk, the studies found no benefit, either.

Again, the studies reviewed relative risk on women who were using synthetic progestin. At the time, the synthetic progestin was given with horse estrogen, which does not represent a female human's estrogen makeup.

But what about the potential brain-protecting aspects of actual human hormones? Is there evidence that using actual human copies of hormones confers brain protection or benefit?

Although multiple links to our environment, diet, lifestyle, and genetics can play a role in brain health, some studies point to hormones as also having a role in brain health. Animal studies have shown estrogen to be brain-protective. And in large studies, certain forms of estrogen have been found to protect against Alzheimer's and dementia.

For the most part, a link between hormone replacement and brain protection is difficult to prove because of the insidious nature of many neurologic disorders. Many brain disease states, such as dementia, can be pretty ambiguous; symptoms of brain disease present more or less similarly to what's commonly referred to as "old age."

Alzheimer's is a terrifying disease, and the definitive diagnosis is to see if there are certain plaques in the brain at autopsy, which obviously does not help a living person struggling with what are likely the effects of the disease.

While it can be diagnosed as likely to be occurring in a person, Alzheimer's is what is known as a "diagnosis of exclusion." When there are memory or other neurological problems, tests such as blood work, X-rays, and psychological analysis are performed to look for depression, infection, chemical alterations, or other problems. When those are ruled out but the person's condition continues to worsen, the doctor can tell with a fair degree of certainty that the disease is Alzheimer's.

With Alzheimer's, a diagnosis is important for planning. If someone is losing memory because of depression, an antidepressant may help. But if it is Alzheimer's, the family can start making plans for what to do with the person because Alzheimer's is a progressively worsening disease.

Before I go on, let me explain that we're still learning about the link between hormones and the brain. So the information I'm presenting here is not as clear-cut as some of the other, more time-tested topics that I've discussed in previous chapters. It is cutting-edge, evidence-based medicine, but not to a point that it can clearly guide clinical decisions.

A risk factor for Alzheimer's disease is linked to the abrupt loss of hormones when a woman goes through menopause. Estrogen and progesterone have historically been the hormones studied in menopause, so much of the data is focused on those two. Testosterone levels do not mirror estrogen in menopause. Unless there is a surgery where the ovaries are removed, testosterone tends to fall in a subtler fashion.

Animal studies have shown that blocking androgens tends to lead to Alzheimer's-like plaques building up in the brain.

However, studies looking at sex hormone levels in women and men have shown that those with Alzheimer's had lower circulating sex hormones than age-matched controls. Again, that does not prove a cause. It could be that lower hormones are a risk factor for Alzheimer's, or perhaps Alzheimer's leads to less activity and therefore, fewer hormones. But it has also been found that hormone depletion occurs before the onset of Alzheimer's symptoms. So it may very well be a contributor.

The problem is that other studies have shown that Alzheimer's patients had similar testosterone and estrogen levels to aged-matched controls. A meta-analysis of numerous studies suggested statistically uncertain evidence of a link between low sex steroids and Alzheimer's. The meta-analysis also found that SHBG tended to be elevated in patients with Alzheimer's disease. When SHBG is elevated, the free-circulating sex hormones are depressed, which may contribute to the mixed findings.

All told, there seems to be a link between either decreased sex steroids or decreased free-circulating sex steroids and the development of Alzheimer's.

But again, does that prove causation? One study showed that diminished sex hormones preceded the symptoms of Alzheimer's, but an Alzheimer's diagnosis is typically made after a slow downhill path of dementia. There is not a clear starting point.

Let's look more closely at a few studies. A November 2002 article in the *Journal of the American Medical Association* discussed an observational study in Utah that was performed to evaluate whether HRT influenced the development of Alzheimer's disease.

The study assessed 5,677 elderly individuals for dementia and Alzheimer's. Again, while there is no definitive diagnosis of Alzheimer's prior to an autopsy, doctors who specialize in the disease are 90 percent accurate to eventual autopsy findings.

The women in the study who used HRT throughout their life or for greater than ten years had less than half the rate of Alzheimer's disease as did non-HRT users. The finding, however, was only in women who started HRT early; there was no evidence that HRT would be beneficial once dementia or Alzheimer's has started.

A later meta-analysis looked at whether HRT could reduce risk of Alzheimer's disease. The paper, published in a 2009 issue of *Frontiers in Neuroendocrinology*, reviewed 390 scientific articles and found that it seemed possible that HRT could prove preventive but that, to date, there was no definitive proof.

In the WHI trials, it was noted specifically that starting HRT later in life (over age sixty-five) definitely did not prevent dementia, and there was a possibility that starting it for the first time at that age could even trigger a trend toward dementia. Again, that finding represents the age bias that existed in the WHI trials.

The bottom line is that there is insufficient evidence to suggest that HRT causes or protects against dementia and Alzheimer's. Why is there so little evidence? Because most studies do not go on for more than a few years, and the age of menopause is typically the late forties or early fifties, whereas Alzheimer's is typically diagnosed at or after age sixty-five. Additionally, it has only been a little over a decade since it was discovered that the "HRT of the day" was not ideal and the nation began switching back to more human-like hormones. So the data is still coming out. There is abundant evidence that even synthetic hormones, when started at the onset or near the onset of menopause and taken in the short term or long term, do not cause dementia or Alzheimer's. There appears to be a link between brain protection and long-term use, and there is stronger evidence for natural hormone replacement being brain-protective.

• •

Sue B: Relief in Two Weeks

When Sue B. entered her midforties without any health issues, she considered herself extremely lucky. Then slight changes began creeping in: night sweats, sleeplessness, brain fog, fatigue. "I attributed the changes to normal aging," she said. "But when the night sweats eventually graduated into full-blown hot flashes, I thought, *This can't be menopause, can it?*"

When the list of symptoms continued to grow, Sue knew she had to look for a solution. She initially tried low-dose birth-control pills, hormonal patches, and herbal supplements, but nothing worked. Then she began reading articles on bioidentical hormones. When she found a number of studies that supported using bioidentical hormones as part of hormone replacement therapy, she opted to give them a try.

She visited Allure Medical Spa, where her blood work revealed she was a good candidate for testosterone pellets. "Within two weeks my symptoms were alleviated," she said. "I finally started sleeping again and was able to overcome my slow-to-start mornings. My mental fogginess disappeared and I felt alive again."

Soon thereafter, Sue was motivated to lose the extra twenty pounds she had accumulated, which helped her regain her youthful energy. "Using bioidenticals was the best choice for my hormones, health, and happiness," she said. "Thank you, Dr. Mok!"

• •

Healthy Young Women

Briefly, let me talk about hormones in the nonelderly—in other words, people young enough to have little to no risk of dementia.

A study was conducted at Utrecht University on female students ages eighteen to thirty-five who were not on HRT. The subjects were given a series of memory and cognitive tests and were tested for a baseline. Then the women were given testosterone supplementation and, after about four to six hours, memory was improved, and the women were tested with a vaginal pulse amplitude to verify vaginal response as well.

What they found was *the women had better memory after being supplemented with testosterone.*

What does this prove? On a research level, it may serve as a stepping stone. For me, it offers a chance to share with my female employees (about two hundred at the time of this writing) that "in the book, we pointed out that testosterone makes you smarter!"

Hormones and Migraines

I would be remiss if I did not discuss migraines in a book on menopause.

Migraines are vascular headaches that are more frequent in women than men. Migraines do tend to have hormonal connection and peak between ages thirty-five and forty-five, which is typically the premenopausal time in a woman's life.

The Dayton study, which I mentioned in chapter 2, was designed to determine breast cancer rates in women on testosterone pellets or on testosterone plus an estrogen-blocker pellet. The women had a history of significant migraines, and they had symptoms of hormone deficiency but were not necessarily in menopause.

There were twenty-seven women with significant headaches in the study, and they rated the intensity of the headaches as a three or four on a scale of zero (no pain) to four (severe pain).

About six months after pellet insertion, 74 percent of the women reported a severity of zero, meaning that their headaches were gone. These were women who suffered from headaches at least once a month, and most had them more frequently.

Hormones and Mood

There have been numerous studies and reports on the positive effects of testosterone on mood, a sense of vigor, and decreased fatigue. Many of the studies assessing mood were also studies looking at other benefits of testosterone therapy in women. The question researchers wanted to answer was "Why? Why does testosterone, with or without estrogen, seem to improve mood and well-being in women?"

A study published in Sweden by a department of clinical neuroscience in cooperation with a department of obstetrics and gynecology looking to answer that question started with two facts:

- Serotonin is a chemical in the brain that is clearly linked to depression and anxiety.

- It is one of a group of neurotransmitters, meaning chemicals that the brain uses for perception.

Selective serotonin reuptake inhibitors (SSRIs) are FDA-approved drugs to treat mood disorders such as depression. Examples of SSRIs are Paxil®, Zoloft®, Prozac®, Lexapro®, and Celexa®. They selectively block the reuptake of serotonin to the brain to improve mood from a depressed state.

Hormones seem to play a role in mood. Women are more likely to experience significant mood alterations at times of significant hormone fluctuations, including premenstrual, postpartum, and menopause.

Serotonin is a neurotransmitter that is clearly linked to mood, and significant fluctuations of hormones are linked to mood disorders. But are they related directly or by chance? Prior studies were not designed well enough to determine if there was a link, but they laid the groundwork for this Swedish study to be able to be carried out.

In the study, positron emission tomography (PET) was used to measure serotonin activity in women whose ovaries and uterus were removed for various reasons. The women were not on HRT.

PET is a type of medical scan that can, among other things, measure serotonin activity in various areas of the brain. In depressed patients, PET scans can see that there is less serotonin active in the part of the brain that controls mood. A baseline MRI was used to precisely identify the mood areas of the brain, and the PET was used to overlay serotonin activity in the corresponding areas.

Because of the well-documented effect on sex hormones on sexuality, mood, and well-being, participants in the study were first administered estrogen alone, and then three months later, estrogen plus testosterone. Progesterone was not used because the women did not have ovaries. Researchers measured serotonin activity at baseline, after administration of estrogen alone, and after administration of estrogen plus testosterone.

The women had improvements in both mood and well-being in the estrogen-only as well as the estrogen-plus-testosterone treatment periods. Additionally, verbal fluency improved in only the estrogen-plus-testosterone group.

There were alterations in serotonin activity in various regions of the brain, particularly in the limbic system, which controls mood, memory, habits, and more. Specific areas of altered serotonin included the hypothalamus, cingulate cortex, hippocampus, thalamus, amygdala, and occipital cortex. These are all structures located at the center and rear of the brain that involve involuntary activities rather than active cognitive or intentional thought.

The bottom line of this study is that the mechanism for the improvement of depression and mood disorders with hormone replacement is a little closer to being clarified. It also gives some explanation as to why women with more severe depression who are taking SSRI drugs do better if they are also on hormone replacement.

The study results don't suggest that hormone replacement with either estrogen or testosterone will treat or cure depression, but they do offer insight into the question: "Why does testosterone, with or without estrogen, seem to improve mood and well-being in women?"

Other studies have looked at whether hormones could be used to treat more serious mood disorders. A paper published in 2014 in London looked at the severity of depression in women. In the study, more than two hundred women were treated with estrogen (transdermal or pellets), and most were also treated with testosterone (gel or implant).

The severity of the depression was significant: 71 percent had been on antidepressant medications, 12 percent were treated with inpatient mental therapy, 3.8 percent had received electroconvulsive therapy, and 14 percent had attempted suicide.

The study was unblinded and observational, meaning that there was no placebo and that participants and doctors both knew what treatment was being administered. So there were some inherent limitations that could be argued, particularly if the results were not substantial.

The follow-up results were that 34 percent felt cured of their depression, another 56 percent felt much better, and only 10 percent saw small or no change.

Those were substantial results. Not many drugs are 90 percent effective, particularly for something as troubling as depression, suicide, and mood disturbance.

• •

The Winning Edge

- Women in menopause or perimenopause must understand that healthy hormone levels are brain- and mood-protective.
- Natural hormone replacement appears to be brain-protective.
- Studies have shown that long-term use of HRT does not cause Alzheimer's but potentially can reduce the risk by up to 50 percent.
- Hormone replacement is linked to less depression and better mood.

• •

Chapter 7

AGING AND LONGEVITY

There is a lot of interest in the use of hormone placement as an anti-aging therapy. But can HRT actually prolong a woman's life?

A problem with trying to find out whether hormone placement therapy adds to longevity is the very fact or nature of that kind of study. We need evidence-based medicine in order to answer these kinds of questions, and very long-term studies need to be performed to assess the effects of certain medications on mortality rates.

The situation is confounded by the fact that in the decades it takes to determine whether something prolongs life, therapeutics will change, making slight changes in direction, medications, or doses based on current information.

However, if we already know that maintenance of youthful hormones confers protection against premature death, wouldn't that also seem to answer the question: "If natural hormones are anti-aging, then can hormone replacement also confer protection against aging?"

A 2015 analysis in Belgium attempted to answer that question. Researchers in the study looked at three different published papers on studies using hormone replacement and controls. The studies looked at both men and women and at the hormone replacements that were being used at the time.

The analysis found that testosterone supplementation in men with late-onset decline in testosterone levels increased survival rate by about 10 percent at five years, compared to men who did not receive testosterone placement. The same study also found that estrogen replacement in women likely increased survival by 2.6 percent at five years, compared to women who took no supplements at all.

In reality, much has been said, thought, or assumed about hormone replacement and longevity. It would seem—based on the countless studies that have been done, including a number of which I've discussed in the previous chapters—that since hormone replacement can protect against breast cancer, potentially reduce cardiac risk, reduce fractures, and maintain mood and cognitive function, that HRT must also be able to extend life. While that may be true, there are no real, definitive answers, and making such a claim is just guesswork or speculation.

There is a medical board and certification process through the American Academy of Anti-Aging Medicine. I was a member of the organization, received certification, and was even a board examiner at one time, where I verbally tested other physicians' knowledge.

Ten years ago, I attended a lecture at one of the group's meetings in which the speaker pointed out that with HRT, "The science points to health benefits, and with proper nutrition, exercise, and replacement of deficient hormones, we may not have a significant impact on extending life, but we do see an extension of the period of healthiness." He termed the success with HRT as "health span," as opposed to "life span."

That's really what I'm talking about with HRT. *Isn't it worthwhile to reduce diabetes, heart disease, cancers, and dementia, even if you don't live longer?*

Of course it is. And those conditions can be studied pretty easily in humans. Life span is a very complex object to study. Death may come years to decades after the development of disease. So it's true to say that hormone replacement can benefit your health, even though we do not yet know if hormone optimization can actually extend your life.

As we discussed earlier, in a long-term study with natural hormone replacement, when taken beyond ten years, the rate of fatal heart attacks is reduced by 70 percent (and heart attacks are the leading causes of death in women) and all-cause mortality is also reduced. That means there is less death during the time of the study. But we don't really know what happens beyond the sixteen years of that study. It's very likely that because there were fewer deaths, the women lived longer than the study period (and they obviously lived longer than the untreated women, who had a higher death rate). But "anti-aging" is still a description of intent; we will all still age.

Showing Your Age

Can hormones make you look or feel younger? Obviously, if you have less disease, you can look and feel younger. Hormones can make you feel more sexual, which is associated with feeling young and alive. There are also beneficial effects on weight and body composition.

So just what can HRT do for your physical appearance as you age?

The effect of hormones, particular estrogens in women, is very well-known in dermatology. A study in Austria sought to determine the skin anti-aging effects of estrogen on the skin of middle-aged and older women. Estrogens are known to have a beneficial effect against acne, and this is why many women develop acne while going through menopause. Estrogens also improve vascularization and moisture content of the skin and have a beneficial effect on the elastin in skin.

In the study, women either took a placebo or took estradiol and estriol. Again, estradiol is the dominant estrogen in adult women, and estriol is the estrogen abundant during pregnancy. The study evaluated the effect of estrogen replacement on the facial skin of women averaging fifty-eight years old.

After a few months, there was noticeable wrinkle improvement and reduction in pore size in about 80 percent of the women on estradiol. The majority those who took estriol (more than 90 percent) saw fewer wrinkles, better vascularization, and smaller pores in as few as six weeks. Skin moisture content also went up significantly with both estrogens, leading to a healthy glow. And there were no adverse effects.

Another study using the same estrogens evaluated elasticity, firmness of the skin, wrinkle depth, and amount of collagen fibers. In this study, both compounds were highly effective in preventing or treating skin aging, and there was a notable increase in type III collagen fibers (a fibrous protein in the body's tissues).

There's a common fear that because men develop male pattern baldness, replacement of testosterone in women might lead to scalp hair loss. A study published in 2011 looked at the issue of female pattern hair loss, evaluating testosterone replacement therapy for women in menopause to determine if androgen or testosterone replacement would improve or worsen the issue. About a quarter of women in menopause suffer from female pattern hair loss.

The study, which used testosterone pellets, found that about 70 percent of the women developed increased scalp hair growth and thickness; the rest had no change in scalp hair. No one in the study observed acceleration of hair loss with testosterone replacement.

Bones and Muscle

It is well-known that hormone replacement is protective against osteoporosis bone loss in women in menopause.

A study looked at the response of muscles to exercise in two groups of women, with one taking a placebo and the other taking hormone replacement. Researchers performed laboratory analysis and muscle biopsies after study participants exercised. The study was designed to see if HRT protected muscles against permanent damage when provoked with exercise.

Researchers found that women on HRT had protection against muscle damage, even with maximal exercise effort.

Another study evaluated the use of testosterone in women with oophorectomies, women who no longer had their ovaries. The study looked at sexual activity and desire as well as strength and physical ability. As I discussed in chapter 3, sexual activity increases in most women taking testosterone replacement. This study was no different: Women taking testosterone replacement had sexual activity 2.7 times per week more than women taking nothing. But women on testosterone replacement also had improved lean (fat-free) body mass and improved exercise parameters without adverse effects.

While it really cannot be said that hormone replacement is "anti-aging," as is often claimed, it can be said that hormone replacement protects against many aspects of normal aging. Long-term hormone replacement can reduce fatal heart attacks by over 70 percent and can reduce risks of breast cancer by approximately 70 percent. Hormone replacement can improve sexuality and mood and supports healthy skin and bones. Those attributes may define "anti-aging." However, the medical community tends to look down on the term "anti-aging," as scientific studies typically do not last a human lifetime, and therefore there is no real scientific evidence that hormone replacement is "anti-aging."

• •

The Winning Edge

- There is controversy in the medical community as to whether hormone replacement should be called "anti-aging therapy."
- HRT can protect against muscle damage, even with maximal exercise effort. HRT can also give you thicker hair, fewer wrinkles, and more youthful, glowing skin.
- Hormones do not stop aging. They cannot prevent death or fully prevent disease. But the typical conditions associated with aging, such as cancer, heart disease, weight gain, mood disorders, Alzheimer's, decreased sexuality, skin conditions, and bone and muscle loss tend to occur more often in menopause, and hormone replacement offers some degree of protection.
- Hormone replacement, done right, can delay or lower the risks of developing the conditions and diseases associated with aging.
- There is no stopping nature, but individuals can affect their own health.

• •

Conclusion

THE IDEAL HORMONE
REPLACEMENT PARADIGM

The phrase "the practice of medicine" means that medicine is ever-changing. Unfortunately, it's a field bound by rigid rules that can lead to the inability to adapt to new information and seek out the best individual options.

The best we can do as medical professionals is to work within guidelines, knowing that as viable scientific information presents itself in the future, the guidelines will be adapted to continually offer patients the most appropriate treatments available.

That said, here is where we stand today with hormone replacement therapies used for treating menopausal symptoms.

Menopause is a fact of life, as is aging. But "aging gracefully" can mean that a woman has options for avoiding or reducing the risk for obesity, heart disease, breast cancer, diabetes, Alzheimer's, hair loss, saggy skin, and decreased sexuality and can even reduce the risk of dying of a heart attack. These options should include lifestyle choices such as a healthy diet and exercise, positively influencing community and family, learning, being open-minded, and being generous with talent and resources.

But to be able do all those things requires *treating menopause* like any other treatable condition.

There are detractors of the treatment of menopause. Some people would suggest that women should let nature take its course, that menopause is just part of aging. It is. But women are living longer, more engaged, healthier lives, and they want the second half of their life to be as fulfilling as the first half.

As I've said, discounting the routine treatment of menopause and ovarian failure with hormone replacement is as absurd as discounting the treatment of hypertension because "it's a normal part of aging." Hypertension is no longer ignored because the outcome of untreated hypertension is so solidly established. The outcomes of ovarian failure or removal are solidly established as well. Heart disease, breast cancer, obesity, osteoporosis, mood disorder, and other such outcomes are at least partly reduced or prevented with modern hormone replacement.

A Visit to Allure

Perhaps the best way for me to help you better understand what I mean by "aging gracefully" is to share with you what it's like to visit us at Allure. "Allure" is what we affectionately call our Allure Medical Spa practice located in various locations around Southeastern Michigan.

Once here, you will be greeted by a member of our First Impression Team, who will give you a tour of our office. You will be introduced to your medical assistant, who will ask you some questions about your life, including your family, hobbies, and experiences. We want to get to know you and to know what's important to you.

Then the medical assistant will ask you what main qualifications you look for in a doctor. She will want to know if you are more of a detail person or a bottom-line one. She will ask you questions about your values as well as your concerns.

Then she will give you a questionnaire to fill out. The questionnaire is broken up into various hormone deficiency questions, and your medical assistant can explain to you which questions line up to each deficiency.

On your first visit, we also order blood work: a hormone panel. We use your blood work to confirm or deny what a clinician believes to be your current needs based on the conversation you had with the medical assistant. We believe the best method is to listen to you to understand your symptoms and then use your blood work and tests to confirm the potential diagnosis.

One of my early mentors, Brian Liska, DO, taught me, "When all else fails, ask the patient." His motto is a reminder of some of the primary lessons I learned while in medical school: Medicine is about a patient's history and a physical examination, and laboratory tests are only 10 percent of the overall diagnosis and are used to confirm what the doctor suspects or to question the doctor's judgment. So blood work and tests are in our tool bag, but communication is our key tool for diagnosing patients.

On your first visit, a doctor or nurse practitioner will also talk to you about your medical history and will perform a physical examination. She will also go over your concerns and your symptoms and will ultimately have a look at your blood-work results to help in determining the best course of action for you.

Treatment by Allure

Depending on your needs, here are common treatments administered by Allure:

Perimenopause—For women who are still having periods but are beginning to have menopause symptoms, we generally start with a testosterone pellet, which is implanted in your buttocks. We start by cleaning your skin and injecting an anesthetic to numb the area. A small slit is made in your skin, which of course, you won't feel. Then we insert a rice-sized pellet of testosterone. The slit is so small that a stitch is not needed; we simply apply a small bandage that you later remove.

There are no restrictions and no downtime following the pellet insertion.

You will also likely be given natural progesterone tablets or cream to apply to your skin, per instructions.

Early menopause—For women who have had no period for a year and have symptoms of menopause, we perform the same procedure as for perimenopause women. Again, menopause is a condition where the ovaries fail or have been removed. However, in addition to testosterone, women in early menopause may be given one-tenth as much estrogen. The ten-to-one ratio of testosterone to estrogen mimics the hormone balance of young, healthy women.

Generally, it takes about two weeks for the symptoms of menopause to subside. The pellets last about two and a half to three months the first time they are administered. Subsequent doses tend to last about three to five months.

Progesterone is also given, usually as a daily pill.

Late menopause—Currently, there is less need for estrogen, and treatment is a little simpler. At this point, it's just a matter of getting a testosterone pellet placed every three to five months. The treatment is a little like getting your ovaries working again.

We used to track laboratory values when we were using creams and pills. With pellets, the levels are so consistent that the lab work is more or less useless, so adjustments of dosage are based on symptoms. Again, as my mentor Dr. Brian Liska said, "When all else fails, ask the patient."

Baseline labs can help lay the foundation, and we do follow-up blood work from time to time. But relying on blood tests can be generally misleading.

Most women in our practice who initiate natural hormone replacement intend to continue for the rest of their lives. It doesn't mean you have to, but the evidence shows that the longer you're on treatment, the better. There is no reason to discontinue for health reasons.

There are numerous reasons to replace youthful hormones in women entering or in menopause, not the least of which is improved quality of life.

The focus of this book is to tell you the real story. My job is to read the medical literature and to explain it for you to understand. I use data, science, and facts to get to the point. This approach has helped my career to evolve from treating acute disease and trauma to prevention and health maintenance. It is still evolving, as I transition into more of a leadership and mentoring role to the doctors, physician assistants, nurse practitioners, and the amazing support staff who comprise the Allure team.

When I wrote this chapter, I had on my desk a note from our local metropolitan newspaper, the *Detroit Free Press*, that we were rated in the Top 100 Places to Work in Michigan. And we were just awarded, by *Crain's* business magazine, the honor of being among the "75 Coolest Places to Work."

What that means for you is that a visit to Allure is like being welcomed by family. When you come see us, you'll meet with people who are focused on having an impact on our community and who are committed to training, adapting, and accommodating.

The reason we exist is "to bring out the person you were meant to be." For me, it is about being a leader in HRT and improving people's lives. For others on the team, it is about growing and helping people. Our reason for existing is about

SYMPTOMS OF MENOPAUSE

✓ hot flashes
✓ sweating
✓ sleep problems
✓ moodiness
✓ irritability/anxiety
✓ fatigue
✓ joint and muscle pain
✓ bladder control issues
✓ decreased sexual desire, activity, and satisfaction
✓ decreased thickness and fullness of scalp hair
✓ decreased bone density
✓ memory loss
✓ vaginal dryness

both our staff and our customers. We are a giving, charitable office, and we intend to give more. And our staff is constantly learning and growing.

We have specific core values that we expect from our staff. These are things we are willing to take a financial loss to preserve, and we are willing to terminate members of the team who do not embrace them.

The parent company of my multidivision practice is Allure Medical Spa. Our brand promise is "Excellence in Service, Respect People's Time, and Outstanding Results." We will do whatever it takes to deliver to you our brand promise. It is truly our pleasure to serve you.

Sincerely,

Dr. Charles Mok

For an appointment with us, call Allure Medical Spa at 586-992-8300 or visit us at AllureMedicalSpa.com.

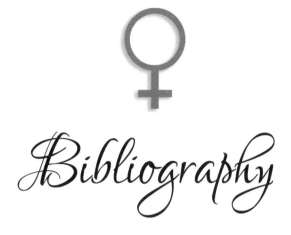

Bibliography

INTRODUCTION

Abdi, Fatemeh, Hamid Mobedi, Nariman Mosaffa, Mahrokh Dolatian, and Fahimeh Ramezani Tehrani. "Hormone Therapy for Relieving Postmenopausal Vasomotor Symptoms: A Systematic Review." *Archives of Iranian Medicine* 19, no. 2 (February 2016): 141–146.

Glaser, Rebecca and Constantine Dimitrakakis. "Testosterone therapy in women: Myths and misconceptions." *Maturitas* 74 (2013): 230–234.

Hargrove, Joel T., Wayne S. Maxson, Anne Colston Wentz, and Lonnie S. Burnett. "Menopausal Hormone Replacement Therapy With Continuous Daily Oral Micronized Estradiol and Progesterone." *Obstetrics & Gynecology* 73, no. 4 (April 1989): 606–612.

Hersh, Adam L., Marcia L. Stefanick, and Randall S. Stafford. "National use of postmenopausal hormone therapy: annual trends and response to recent evidence." *Journal of the American Medical Association* 291, no. 1 (January 20014): 47–53. doi:10.1001/jama.291.1.47.

MacLennan, A. H., A. W. Taylor, and D. H. Wilson. "Hormone therapy use after the Women's Health Initiative." *Climacteric* 7, no. 1 (2004): 138–142. doi: 10.1080/13697130410001713733.

Manson, JoAnn E., Rowan T. Chlebowski, Marcia L. Stefanick, Aaron K. Aragaki, Jacques E. Rossouw, Ross L. Prentice, Garnet Anderson et al. "The Women's Health Initiative Hormone Therapy Trials: Update and Overview of Health Outcomes During the Intervention and Post-Stopping Phases." *Journal of the American Medical Association* 310, no. 13 (October 2, 2013): 1353–1368. doi:10.1001/jama.2013.278040.

Shapiro, Samuel. "Risks of estrogen plus progestin therapy: a sensitivity analysis of findings in the Women's Health Initiative randomized controlled trial." *Climacteric* 6 (2003): 302–310.

Shapiro, Samuel. "The Million Women Study: potential biases do not allow uncritical acceptance of the data." *Climacteric* 7 (2004): 3–7.

Tutera, Gino. "Marked Reduction of Breast, Endometrial, and Ovarian Cancer in Users of Bio-Identical Estradiol and Testosterone Subcutaneous Pellets." *Maturitas* 63, no. 1 (2009).

WHI Steering Committee. "Effects of Conjugated Equine Estrogen in Postmenopausal Women With Hysterectomy." *Journal of the American Medical Association* 291, no. 14 (April 14, 2014): 1701–1712.

Writing Group for the Women's Health Initiative Investigators. "Risks and Benefits of Estrogen Plus Progestin in Healthy Postmenopausal Women." *Journal of the American Medical Association* 288, no. 3 (July 17, 2002): 321–333.

CHAPTER 2

Bankhead, Charles. "ASCO Breast: Implants May Quell Hormone Deficiency." *MedPage Today* (October 4, 2010).

Cordina-Duverger, Emilie, Thérèse Truong, Antoinette Anger, Marie Sanchez, Patrick Arveux, Pierre Kerbrat, and Pascal Guénel. "Risk of Breast Cancer by Type of Menopausal Hormone Therapy: a Case-Control Study among Post-Menopausal Women in France." *PLOS ONE* 8, no. 11 (November 2013): 1–9. doi:10.1371/journal.pone.0078016.

Dew, J. E., B. G. Wren, and J. A. Eden. "A cohort study of topical vaginal estrogen therapy in women previously treated for breast cancer." *Climacteric* 6 (2003): 45–52.

Dimitrakakis, Constantine, David Zava, Spyros Marinopoulos, Alexandra Tsigginou, Aris Antsaklis, and Rebecca Glaser. "Low salivary testosterone levels in patients with breast cancer." *BMC Cancer* (2010): 1–8. doi:10.1186/1471-2407-10-547.

Dimitrakakis, Constantine, Jian Zhou, Jie Wang, Alain Belanger, Fernand LaBrie, Clara Cheng, Douglas Powell, and Carolyn Bondy. "A physiologic role for testosterone in limiting estrogenic stimulation of the breast." *Menopause* 10, no. 4 (2003): 292–298. doi: 10.1097/01.GME.0000055522.67459.89.

Dimitrakakis, Constantine, Jian Zhou, and Carolyn A. Bondy. "Androgens and mammary growth and neoplasia." *Fertility and Sterility* 77, no. 4 (April 2002): S26–S33.

Dimitrakakis, Constantine, Robert A. Jones, Aiyi Liu, and Carolyn A. Bondy. "Breast cancer incidence in postmenopausal women using testosterone in addition to usual hormone therapy." *Menopause* 11, no. 5 (2004): 531–535. doi: 10.1097/01.GME.0000119983.48235.D3.

Fournier, Agnes, Franco Berrino, and Francoise Clavel-Chapelon. "Unequal risks for breast cancer associated with different hormone replacement therapies: results from the E3N cohort study." *Breast Cancer Research and Treatment* 107 (2008): 103–111. doi: 10.1007/s10549-007-9523-x.

Glaser, Rebecca L., Anne E. York, and Constantine Dimitrakakis. "Efficacy of subcutaneous testosterone on menopausal symptoms in breast cancer survivors." Abstract. Breast Cancer Symposium. (2014).

Glaser, Rebecca L. and Constantine Dimitrakakis. "Rapid response of breast cancer to neoadjuvant intramammary testosterone-anastrozole therapy: neoadjuvant hormone therapy in breast cancer." *Menopause* 21, no. 6 (2013): 1–6. doi: 10.1097/gme.0000000000000096.

Glaser, Rebecca L. and Constantine Dimitrakakis. "Reduced breast cancer incidence in women treated with subcutaneous testosterone, or testosterone with anastrozole: A prospective, observational study."*Maturitas* 76 (2013): 342–349.

Glaser, Rebecca L. and Constantine Dimitrakakis. "Testosterone and breast cancer prevention." Maturitas 82 (2015): 290–294.

Glaser, Rebecca L. "Subcutaneous Testosterone-Anastrozole Therapy in Breast Cancer Survivors." (2010 ASCO Breast Cancer Symposium). PowerPoint presentation. 26 slides.

Hofling, Marie, Angelica Linden Hirschberg, Lambert Skoog, Edneia Tani, Torsten Hagerstrom, and Bo von Schoultz. "Testosterone inhibits estrogen/progestogen-induced breast cell proliferation in postmenopausal women." *Menopause* 14, no. 2 (2007): 1–8. doi: 10.1097/01.gme.0000232033.92411.51.

Lyytinen, Heli, Eero Pukkala, and Olavi Ylikorkala. "Breast Cancer Risk in Postmenopausal Women Using Estrogen-Only Therapy." *Obstetrics & Gynecology* 108, no. 6 (December 2006): 1354–1360.

Magnusson, Cecilia, Lars Holmberg, Torgny Norden, Anders Lindgren, and Ingemar Persson. "Prognostic characteristics in breast cancers after hormone replacement therapy." *Breast Cancer Research and Treatment* 38 (1996): 325–334.

Million Women Study Collaborators. "Breast cancer and hormone-replacement therapy in the Million Women Study." *The Lancet* 362 (August 9, 2003): 419–427.

Natrajan, Puthugramam K. and R. Don Gambrell, Jr. "Estrogen replacement therapy in patients with early breast cancer." *American Journal of Obstetrics & Gynecology* 187, no. 2 (2002): 289–295. doi:10.1067/mob.2002.125999.

Plu-bureau, G., M. G. Le, J. C. Thalabard, R. Sitruk-Ware, and P. Mauvais-Jarvis. "Percutaneous Progesterone Use and Risk of Breast Cancer: Results from a French Cohort Study of Premenopausal Women with Benign Breast Disease." *Cancer Detection and Prevention* 23, no. 4 (1999): 290–296.

Somboonporn, Woraluk and Susan R. Davis. "Postmenopausal testosterone therapy and breast cancer risk." *Maturitas* 49 (2004) 267–275. doi:10.1016/j.maturitas.2004.06.020.

Somboonporn, Woraluk and Susan R. Davis. "Testosterone Effects on the Breast: Implications for Testosterone Therapy for Women." *Endocrine Reviews* 25, no. 3 (June 2004): 373–388. doi: 10.1210/er.2003-0016.

Tutera, Gino. "Marked Reduction of Breast, Endometrial, and Ovarian Cancer in Users of Bio-Identical Estradiol and Testosterone Subcutaneous Pellets." *Maturitas* 63, no. 1 (2009).

Writing Group for the Women's Health Initiative Investigators. "Risks and Benefits of Estrogen Plus Progestin in Healthy

Postmenopausal Women." *Journal of the American Medical Association* 288, no. 3 (July 17, 2002): 321–333.

Zhou, Jian, Siu Ng, O. Adesanya-Famuiya, Kristin Anderson, and Carolyn A. Bondy. "Testosterone inhibits estrogen-induced mammary epithelial proliferation and suppresses estrogen receptor expression." *The FASEB Journal* 14 (September 2004): 1725–1730.

CHAPTER 3

Alexander, Jeanne Leventhal, Krista Kotz, Lorraine Dennerstein, S. Jerome Kutner, Kim Wallen, and Morris Notelovitz. "The effects of postmenopausal hormone therapies on female sexual functioning: a review of double-blind, randomized controlled trials." *The Journal of the North American Menopause Society* 11, no. 6 (2004): 749–765. doi: 10.1097/01. GME.0000142887.31811.97.

Burger, H. G., J. Hailes, M. Menelaus, J. Nelson, B. Hudson, and N. Balazs. "The management of persistent menopausal symptoms with oestradiol–testosterone implants: clinical, lipid and hormonal results." *Maturitas* 6 (1984): 351–358.

Davis, Andra S., Kay Gilbert, Philip Misiowiec, and Barbara Riegel. "Perceived Effects of Testosterone Replacement Therapy in Perimenopausal and Postmenopausal Women: An Internet Pilot Study." *Health Care for Women International* 24 (2003): 831–848. doi: 10 1080/07399330390229902.

Floter, A., J. Nathorst-Böös, K. Carlström, and B. von Schoultz. "Addition of testosterone to estrogen replacement therapy in oophorectomized women: effects on sexuality and well-being." *Climacteric* 5 (2002): 357–365.

Goldstat, Rebecca, Esther Briganti, Jane Tran, Rory Wolfe, and Susan R. Davis. "Transdermal testosterone therapy improves well-being, mood, and sexual function in premenopausal women." *Menopause* 10, no. 5 (2003): 390–398. doi: 10.1097/OI.GME.0000060256.03945.20.

Huang, Grace, Shehzad Basaria, Thomas G. Travison, Matthew H. Ho, Maithili Davda, Norman A. Mazer, Renee Miciek et al. "Testosterone Dose-Response Relationships in Hysterectomized Women with and without Oophorectomy: Effects on Sexual Function, Body Composition, Muscle Performance and Physical Function in a Randomized Trial." *Menopause* 21, no. 6 (June 2014): 612–623. doi:10.1097/GME.0000000000000093.

North American Menopause Society, "The role of testosterone therapy in postmenopausal women: position statement of The North American Menopause Society," *Menopause: The Journal of the North American Menopause Society* 12, no. 5 (September-October 2005):496–511. http://www.ncbi.nlm.nih.gov/pubmed/16145303.

Randolph, Jr., John F., Huiyong Zheng, Nancy E. Davis, Gail A. Greendale, and Sioban D. Harlow. "Masturbation Frequency and Sexual Function Domains Are Associated With Serum

Reproductive Hormone Levels Across the Menopausal Transition." *Journal of Clinical Endocrinology & Metabolism* 100, no. 1 (January 2015): 258–266. doi: 10.1210/jc.2014-1725.

Shifren, Jan L., Glenn D. Braunstein, James A. Simon, Peter R. Casson, John E. Buster, Geoffrey P. Redmond, Regula E. Burki et al. "Transdermal Testosterone Treatment in Women with Impaired Sexual Function after Oophorectomy." *The New England Journal of Medicine* 343, no. 10 (September 2000): 682–688.

Somboonporn, W., S. Davis, M. W. Seif, R. Bell. "Testosterone for peri- and postmenopausal women (Review)." *The Cochrane Library* 1 (2008).

Turna, B., E. Apaydin, B. Semerci, B. Altay, N. Cikili, and O. Nazli. "Women with low libido: correlation of decreased androgen levels with female sexual function index." *International Journal of Impotence Research* 17 (2005): 148–153.

The North American Menopause Society. "The role of testosterone therapy in postmenopausal women: position statement of The North American Menopause Society." *Menopause* 12, no. 5 (2005): 497–511. doi: 10.1097/01.gme.0000177709.65944. b0.

US Food and Drug Administration. "Information on Compounding." Last updated October 17, 2016. http://www.fda. gov/drugs/GuidanceComplianceRegulatoryInformation/ PharmacyCompounding.

Weirman, Margaret E., Wiebke Arlt, Rosemary Basson, Susan R. Davis, Karen K. Miller, Mohammad H. Murad, William Rosner, and Nanette Santoro. "Androgen Therapy in Women: A Reappraisal: An Endocrine Society Clinical Practice Guideline." *Journal of Clinical Endocrinology & Metabolism* 99, no. 10 (October 2014): 3489–3510. doi: 10.1210/jc.2014-2260.

CHAPTER 4

Benn, Marianne, Sidsel Skou Voss, Haya N. Holmegard, Gorm B. Jensen, Anne Tybjærg-Hansen, and Børge G. Nordestgaard. "Extreme Concentrations of Endogenous Sex Hormones, Ischemic Heart Disease, and Death in Women." *Ateriosclerosis, Thrombosis, and Vascular Biology* 35 (2015): 471–477. doi: 10.1161/ATVBAHA.114.304821.

Committee on Gynecologic Practice. "Hormone Therapy and Heart Disease." *Obstetrics & Gynecology* 121, no. 6. (June 2013): 1407–1410.

Dai, Wen, Wang Ming, Yan Li, Hong-yun Zheng, Chuan-dong Wei, Zhao Rui, and Cui Yan. *Archives of Medical Research* 46 (2015): 619–629.

Golden, Sherita Hill, Ann Maguire, Jingzhong Ding, J. R. Crouse, Jane A. Cauley, Howard Zacur, and Moyses Szklo. "Endogenous Postmenopausal Hormones and Carotid Atherosclerosis: A Case-Control Study of the Atherosclerosis Risk in Communities Cohort." *American Journal of Epidemiology* 155, no. 5 (2002): 437–445.

Huang, Grace, Elizabeth Tang, Adam Aakil, Stephan Anderson, Hernan Jara, Maithili Davda, Helene Stroh et al. "Testosterone Dose-Response Relationships With Cardiovascular Risk Markers in Androgen-Deficient Women: A Randomized, Placebo-Controlled Trial." *Journal of Clinical Endocrinology & Metabolism* 99, no. 7 (July 2014): E1287–E1293. doi: 10.1210/jc.2013-4160.

Kaczmarek, Agnieszka, Krzysztof Reczuch, Jacek Majda, Waldemar Banasiak, and Piotr Ponikowski. "The association of lower testosterone level with coronary artery disease in postmenopausal women." *International Journal of Cardiology* 87 (2003): 53–57.

Kotsopoulos, Worboys S., D. Teede, H. McGrath, and B. P. Davis, Sr. "Subcutaneous Testosterone Implant Therapy Improves Endothelium-Dependent and Independent Vasodilation in Postmenopausal Women Already Receiving Oestrogen." *Heart, Lung and Circulation* 9 (2000).

Miyagawa, Koichi, Josef Rosch, Frank Stanczyk, and Kent Hermsmeyer. "Medroxyprogesterone interferes with ovarian steroid protection against coronary vasospasm." *Nature Medicine* 3, no. 3 (March 1997): 324–327.

Mueck, A. O. "Postmenopausal hormone replacement therapy and cardiovascular disease: the value of transdermal estradiol and micronized progesterone." *Climacteric* 15 (2012): 11–17. doi: 10.3109/13697137.2012.669624.

Post, Marinka S., M. Christella, L. G. D. Thomassen, Marius J. van der Mooren, W. Marchien van Baal, Jan Rosing, Peter Kenemans, and Coen D. A. Stehouwer. "Effect of Oral and Transdermal Estrogen Replacement Therapy on Hemostatic Variables Associated With Venous Thrombosis." *Ateriosclerosis, Thrombosis, and Vascular Biology* 23 (2003): 1116–1121. doi: 10.1161/01.ATV.0000074146.36646.C8.

Rosano, Giuseppe M. C., Carolyn M. Webb, Sergio Chierchia, Gian Luigi Morgani, Michele Gabraele, Phillip M. Sarrel, Dominique de Zieglier, and Peter Collins. "Natural Progesterone, but Not Medroxyprogesterone Acetate, Enhances the Beneficial Effect of Estrogen on Exercise-Induced Myocardial Ischemia in Postmenopausal Women." *Journal of the American College of Cardiology* 36, no. 7 (2000): 2154–2159.

Rouver, Wender Nascimento, Nathalie Tristão Banhos Delgado, Jussara Bezerra Menezes, Roger Lyrio Santos, and Margareth Ribeiro Moyses. "Testosterone Replacement Therapy Prevents Alterations of Coronary Vascular Reactivity Caused by Hormone Deficiency Induced by Castration." PLOS ONE 10, no. 8 (August 2015). doi:10.1371/journal.pone.0137111.

Schierbeck, Louise Lind, Lars Rejnmark, Charlotte Landbo Tofteng, Lis Stilgren, Pia Eiken, Leif Mosekilde, Lars Kober, and Jens-Erik Beck Jensen. "Effect of hormone replacement therapy on cardiovascular events in recently postmenopausal women: randomized trial." *British Medical Journal* 345 (October 2012). doi: 10.1136/bmj.e6409.

Sitruk-Ware, R. L. "Hormone therapy and the cardiovascular system: the critical role of progestins." *Climacteric* 6 (2003): 21–28.

Stanczyk, Frank Z., Donna Shoupe, Victoria Nunez, Priscilla Macias-Gonzales, Marcela A. Vijod, and Rogerio A. Lobo. "A randomized comparison of nonoral estradiol delivery in postmenopausal women." *American Journal of Obstetrics & Gynecology* 159, no. 6 (December 1988): 1540–1546.

Thomas, T., J. Rhodin, L. Clark, and A. Garces. "Progestins initiate adverse events of menopausal estrogen therapy." *Climacteric* 6 (2003): 293–301.

US Department of Health and Human Services. "Hormone Replacement Therapy and Heart Disease: The PEPI Trial." NIH Publication No. 95-3277 (August 1995).

Walsh, Brian W., Helena Li, and Frank M. Sacks. "Effects of postmenopausal hormone replacement therapy with oral and transdermal estrogen on high density lipoprotein metabolism." *Journal of Lipid Research* 35 (1994): 2083–2093.

CHAPTER 5

Al-Asmakh, Maha, and Lars Hedin. "Microbiota and the control of blood-tissue barriers." *Tissue Barriers* 3, no. 3 (July/August/September 2015).

Al-Asmakh, Maha, Jan-Bernd Stukenborg, Ahmed Reda, Farhana Anuar, Mona-Lisa Strand, Lars Hedin, Sven Pettersson, and

Olle Söder. "The Gut Microbiota and Developmental Programming of the Testis in Mice." *PLOS ONE* 9, no. 8 (2014). doi:10.1371/journal.pone.0103809.

Annalisa, Noce, Tarantino Alessio, Tsague Djoutsop Claudette, Vasili Erald, De Lorenzo Antonino, and Di Daniele Nicola. "Gut Microbioma Population: An Indicator Really Sensible to Any Change in Age, Diet, Metabolic Syndrome, and Life-Style." *Mediators of Inflammation* (2014). doi:10.1155/2014/901308.

Aragón, Felix, Gabriela Perdigón, and Alejandra de Moreno de LeBlanc. "Modification in the diet can induce beneficial effects against breast cancer." *World Journal of Clinical Oncology* 5, no. 3 (August 2014): 455–464. doi:10.5306/wjco.v5.i3.455.

Balliett, Mary, and Jeanmarie R. Burke. "Changes in anthropometric measurements, body composition, blood pressure, lipid profile, and testosterone in patients participating in a low-energy dietary intervention." *Journal of Chiropractic Medicine* 12 (2013): 3–14. doi:10.1016/j.jcm.2012.11.003.

Beltrán-Barrientos, L. M., A. Hernández-Mendoza, M. J. Torres-Llanez, A. F. González-Córdova, and B. Vallejo-Córdoba. "Invited review: Fermented milk as antihypertensive functional food." J. Dairy Sci. 99 (2016): 4099-4110. doi:10.3168/jds.2015-10054.

Bitoska, Iskra, Branka Krstevska, Tatjana Milenkovic, Slavica Sub-eska-Stratrova, Goran Petrovski, Sasha Jovanovska Mishevska, Irfan Ahmeti, and Biljana Todorova. "Effects of Hormone Replacement Therapy on Insulin Resistance in Postmeno-pausal Diabetic Women." *Open Access Macedonian Journal of Medical Sciences* 4, no. 1 (March 2016): 83–88. doi:10.3889/oamjms.2016.024.

Bull, Matthew J., and Nigel T. Plummer. "Part 1: The Human Gut Microbiome in Health and Disease." *Integrative Medicine* 13, no. 6 (December 2014): 17–22.

Cavallini, Daniela Cardoso Umbelino, Marla Simone Jovenasso Manzoni, Raquel Bedani, Mariana Nougalli Roselino, Larissa Sbaglia Celiberto, Regina Célia Vendramini, Graciela Font de Valdez et al. "Probiotic Soy Product Supplemented with Iso-flavones Improves the Lipid Profile of Moderately Hypercho-lesterolemic Men: A Randomized Controlled Trial." *Nutrients* 8, no. 52 (2016). doi:10.3390/nu8010052.

Chakraborti, Chandra Kanti. "New-found link between microbiota and obesity." *World Journal of Gastrointestinal Pathophysiol-ogy* 6, no. 4 (November 2015): 110–119. doi:10.4291/wjgp.v6.i4.110.

Chen, Jun, Nicholas Chia, Krishna R. Kalari, Janet Z. Yao, Martina Novotna, M. Mateo Paz Soldan, David H. Luckey et al. "Multiple sclerosis patients have a distinct gut microbiota compared to healthy controls." *Scientific Reports* (2016). doi:10.1038/srep28484.

Chmouliovsky, L., F. Habicht, R.W. James, T. Lehmann, A. Campana, and A. Golay. "Beneficial effect of hormone replacement therapy on weight loss in obese menopausal women." *Maturitas* 32 (1999): 147–153.

Cox-York, Kimberly A., Amy M. Sheflin, Michelle T. Foster, Christopher L. Gentile, Amber Kahl, Lauren G. Koch, Steven L. Britton, and Tiffany L. Weir. "Ovariectomy results in differential shifts in gut microbiota in low versus high aerobic capacity rats." *Physiological Reports* 3, no. 8 (2015). doi:10.14814/phy2.12488.

Daniel, Hannelore, Amin Moghaddas Gholami, David Berry, Charles Desmarchelier, Hannes Hahne, Gunnar Loh, Stanislas Mondot et al. "High-fat diet alters gut microbiota physiology in mice." ISME Journal 8 (2014): 295–308. doi:10.1038/ismej.2013.155.

Dominianni, Christine, Rashmi Sinha, James J. Goedert, Zhiheng Pei, Liying Yang, Richard B. Hayes, and Jiyoung Ahn. "Sex, Body Mass Index, and Dietary Fiber Intake Influence the Human Gut Microbiome." PLOS ONE 10, no. 4 (2015). doi:10.1371/journal.pone.0124599.

El-Salhy, Magdy, Tarek Mazzawi, Trygve Hausken, and Jan Gunnar Hatlebakk. "Interaction between diet and gastrointestinal endocrine cells (Review)." *Biomedical Reports* 4 (2016): 651–656. doi:10.3892/br.2016.649.

Erlanson-Albertsson, Charlotte , and Per-Åke Albertsson. "The Use of Green Leaf Membranes to Promote Appetite Control, Suppress Hedonic Hunger and Loose Body Weight." *Plant Foods Hum Nutr* (2015): 281–290. doi:10.1007/ s11130-015-0491-8.

Espeland, Mark A., Marcia L. Stefanick, Donna Kritz-Silverstein, S. Edwin Fineberg, Myron A. Waclawiw, Margaret K. James, and Gail A. Greendale. "Effect of Postmenopausal Hormone Therapy on Body Weight and Waist and Hip Girths." *Journal of Clinical Endocrinology and Metabolism* 82, no. 5 (1997): 1549–1556.

Fernandez-Raudales, Dina, Jennifer L. Hoeflinger, Neal A. Bringe, Stephen B. Cox, Scot E. Dowd, Michael J. Miller, and Elvira Gonzalez de Mejia. "Consumption of different soymilk formulations differentially affects the gut microbiomes of overweight and obese men." *Gut Microbes* 3, no. 6 (2012): 490–500. doi:10.4161/gmic.21578.

Flores, Roberto, Jianxin Shi, Barbara Fuhrman, Xia Xu, Timothy D. Veenstra, Mitchell H. Gail, Pawel Gajer, Jacques Ravel, and James J. Goedert. "Fecal microbial determinants of fecal and systemic estrogens and estrogen metabolites: a cross-sectional study." *Journal of Translational Medicine* 10 (2012): 253. doi:10.1186/1479-5876-10-253.

Fontana, Luigi, and Linda Partridge. "Promoting Health and Longevity through Diet: from Model Organisms to Humans."

Cell 161, no. 1 (March 2015): 106–118. doi:10.1016/j. cell.2015.02.020.

Fuhrman, Barbara J., Heather Spencer Feigelson, Roberto Flores, Mitchell H. Gail, Xia Xu, Jacques Ravel, and James J. Goedert. "Associations of the Fecal Microbiome With Urinary Estrogens and Estrogen Metabolites in Postmenopausal Women." *Journal of Clinical Endocrinology and Metabolism* 99, no. 2 (December 2014): 4632–4640. doi:10.1210/ jc.2014-2222.

García-Gómez, Elizabeth, Bertha González-Pedrajo, and Ignacio Camacho-Arroyo. "Role of Sex Steroid Hormones in Bacterial-Host Interactions." *BioMed Research International* (2013). doi:10.1155/2013/928290.

Goss, A. M., B. E. Darnell, M. A. Brown, R. A. Oster, and B. A. Gower. "Longitudinal associations of the endocrine environment on fat partitioning in postmenopausal women." Obesity 20, no. 5 (May 2012): 939–944. doi:10.1038/oby.2011.362.

Griffin, Julian L., Xinzhu Wang, and Elizabeth Stanley. "Does Our Gut Microbiome Predict Cardiovascular Risk? A Review of the Evidence from Metabolomics." *Circulation: Cardiovascular Genetics* 8, no. 1 (February 2015): 187–191. doi:10.1161/ CIRCGENETICS.114.000219.

Gruber, Doris M., Michael O. Sator, Sylvia Kirchengast, Elmar A. Joura, and Johannes C. Huber. "Effect of percutaneous androgen replacement therapy on body composition and body weight in postmenopausal women." *Maturitas* 29 (1998): 253–259.

Guo, Yanjie, Yane Qi, Xuefei Yang, Lihui Zhao, Shu Wen, Yinhui Liu, and Li Tang. "Association between Polycystic Ovary Syndrome and Gut Microbiota." *PLOS ONE* (April 2016). doi:10.1371/journal.pone.0153196.

Harada, Naoki, Ryo Hanaoka, Hiroko Horiuchi, Tomoya Kitakaze, Takakazu Mitani, Hiroshi Inui, and Ryoichi Yamaji. "Castration influences intestinal microflora and induces abdominal obesity in high-fat diet-fed mice." *Scientific Reports* 6 (2016). doi:10.1038/srep23001.

Haro, Carmen, Oriol A. Rangel-Zúñiga, Juan F. Alcalá-Díaz, Francisco Gómez-Delgado, Pablo Pérez-Martínez, Javier Delgado-Lista, Gracia M. Quintana-Navarro et al. "Intestinal Microbiota Is Influenced by Gender and Body Mass Index." *PLOS ONE* 11, no. 5 (2016). doi:10.1371/journal.pone.0154090.

Jackson, Melinda L., Henry Butt, Michelle Ball, Donald P. Lewis, and Dorothy Bruck. "Sleep quality and the treatment of intestinal microbiota imbalance in Chronic Fatigue Syndrome: A pilot study." *Sleep Science* 8 (2015): 124–133. doi:10.1016/j.slsci.2015.10.001.

Jeffery, Ian B., and Paul W. O'Toole. "Diet-Microbiota Interactions and Their Implications for Healthy Living." *Nutrients* 5 (2013): 234–252. doi:10.3390/nu5010234.

Khalili, Hamed, Ashwin N. Ananthakrishnan, Gauree G. Konijeti, Leslie M. Higuchi, Charles S. Fuchs, James M. Richter, Shelley S. Tworoger, Susan E. Hankinson, and Andrew T. Chan. "Endogenous Levels of Circulating Androgens and Risk of Crohn's Disease and Ulcerative Colitis Among Women: A Nested Case–Control Study from the Nurses' Health Study Cohorts." *Inflammatory Bowel Diseases* 21, no. 6 (June 2015): 1378–1385.

Kim, Eunjung, Dan-Bi Kim, and Jae-Yong Park. "Changes of Mouse Gut Microbiota Diversity and Composition by Modulating Dietary Protein and Carbohydrate Contents: A Pilot Study." *Preventive Nutrition and Food Science* 21, no. 1 (2016): 57–61. doi:10.3746/pnf.2016.21.1.57.

Kobyliak, Nazarii, Oleksandr Virchenko, and Tetyana Falalyeyeva. "Pathophysiological role of host microbiota in the development of obesity." *Nutrition Journal* 15, no. 43 (2016). doi:10.1186/s12937-016-0166-9.

Kritz-Silverstein, Donna, and Elizabeth Barrett-Connor. "Long-term Postmenopausal Hormone Use, Obesity, and Fat Distribution in Older Women." *Journal of the American Medical Association* 275, no. 1 (January 1996): 46–49.

Le Barz, Mélanie, Fernando F. Anhê, Thibaut V. Varin, Yves Desjardins, Emile Levy, Denis Roy, Maria C. Urdaci, André Marette et al. "Probiotics as Complementary Treatment for Metabolic Disorders." *Diabetes & Metabolism Journal* 29 (2015): 291–303. doi:10.4093/dmj.2015.39.4.291.

Liu, Tzu-Wen, Young-Min Park, Hannah D. Holscher, Jaume
    Padilla, Rebecca J. Scroggins, Rebecca Welly, Steven L.
    Britton et al. "Physical Activity Differentially Affects the
    Cecal Microbiota of Ovariectomized Female Rats Selectively
    Bred for High and Low Aerobic Capacity." *PLOS ONE* 10,
    no. 8 (2015). doi:10.1371/journal.pone.0136150.

Lopez-Legarrea, Patricia, Nicholas Robert Fuller, María Angeles
    Zulet, Jose Alfredo Martinez, and Ian Douglas Caterson.
    "The influence of Mediterranean, carbohydrate and high
    protein diets on gut microbiota composition in the treatment
    of obesity and associated inflammatory state." *Asia Pac
    J Clin Nutr* 23, no. 3 (2014): 360–368. doi:10.6133/
    apjcn.2014.23.3.16.

Lyte, Mark, Ashley Chapel, Joshua M. Lyte, Yongfeng Ai, Alexandra
    Proctor, Jay-Lin Jane, and Gregory J. Phillips. "Resistant
    Starch Alters the Microbiota-Gut Brain Axis: Implications
    for Dietary Modulation of Behavior." *PLOS ONE* 11, no. 1
    (2016). doi:10.1371/journal.pone.0146406.

Markle, Janet G. M., Daniel N. Frank, Steven Mortin-Toth,
    Charles E. Robertson, Leah M. Feazel, Ulrike Rolle-Kamp-
    czyk, Martin von Bergen et al. "Sex Differences in the Gut
    Microbiome Drive Hormone-Dependent Regulation of
    Autoimmunity." Science 339 (March 2013): 1084–1088.
    doi:10.1126/science.1233521.

McAllister, Emily J., Nikhil V. Dhurandhar, Scott W. Keith, Louis
    J. Aronne, Jamie Barger, Monica Baskin, Ruth M. Benca et

al. "Ten Putative Contributors to the Obesity Epidemic." *Crit Rev Food Sci Nutr* 49, no. 10 (November 2009): 868–913. doi:10.1080/10408390903372599.

Montelius, Caroline, Daniel Erlandsson, Egzona Vitija, Eva-Lena Stenblom, Emil Egecioglu, and Charlotte Erlanson-Albertsson. "Body weight loss, reduced urge for palatable food and increased release of GLP-1 through daily supplementation with green-plant membranes for three months in overweight women." *Appetite* 81 (2014): 295–304. doi:10.1016/j.appet.2014.06.101.

Montelius, Caroline, Nadia Osman, Björn Weström, Siv Ahrné, Göran Molin, Per-Åke Albertsson, and Charlotte Erlanson-Albertsson. "Feeding spinach thylakoids to rats modulates the gut microbiota, decreases food intake and affects the insulin response." *Journal of Nutritional Science* 2 (2013). doi:10.1017/jns.2012.29.

Mueck, A. O. "Postmenopausal hormone replacement therapy and cardiovascular disease: the value of transdermal estradiol and micronized progesterone." *Climacteric* 15 (2012): 11–17. doi: 10.3109/13697137.2012.669624.

Mulak, Agata, Yvette Taché, and Muriel Larauche. "Sex hormones in the modulation of irritable bowel syndrome." *World Journal of Gastroenterology* 20, no. 10 (March 2014): 2433–2448. doi:10.3748/wjg.v20.i10.2433.

Nettleton, Jodi E., Raylene A. Reimer, and Jane Shearer. "Reshaping the gut microbiota: Impact of low calorie sweeteners and the link to insulin resistance?" *Physiology & Behavior* (2016). doi:10.1016/j.physbeh.2016.04.029.

Oh, Bumjo, Jong Seung Kim, Meera Kweon, Bong-Soo Kim, and In Sil Huh. "Six-week Diet Correction for Body Weight Reduction and Its Subsequent Changes of Gut Microbiota: A Case Report." *Clinical Nutrition Research* 5 (2016): 137–140. doi:10.7762/cnr.2016.5.2.137.

O'Sullivan, Anthony J., Leonie J. Crampton, Judith Freund, and Ken K. Y. Ho. "The Route of Estrogen Replacement Therapy Confers Divergent Effects on Substrate Oxidation and Body Composition in Postmenopausal Women." *J Clin Invest* 102, no. 5 (September 1998): 1035–1040.

Poutahidis, Theofilos, Alex Springer, Tatiana Levkovich, Peimin Qi, Bernard J. Varian, Jessica R. Lakritz, Yassin M. Ibrahim et al. "Probiotic Microbes Sustain Youthful Serum Testosterone Levels and Testicular Size in Aging Mice." *PLOS ONE* 9, no. 1 (2014). doi:10.1371/journal.pone.0084877.

Scher, Jose U., Carles Ubeda, Alejandro Artacho, Mukundan Attur, Sandrine Isaac, Soumya M. Reddy, Shoshana Marmon et al. "Decreased Bacterial Diversity Characterizes an Altered Gut Microbiota in Psoriatic Arthritis and Resembles Dysbiosis of Inflammatory Bowel Disease." *Arthritis & Rheumatology* 67, no. 1 (January 2015): 128–139. doi:10.1002/art.38892.

Schwabe, Robert, and Christian Jobin. "The microbiome and cancer." *Nature Reviews Cancer* 13, no. 11 (November 2013): 800–812. doi:10.1038/nrc3610.

Sjögren, Klara, Cecilia Engdahl, Petra Henning, Ulf H. Lerner, Valentina Tremaroli, Marie K. Lagerquist, Fredrik Bäckhed, and Claes Ohlsson. "The Gut Microbiota Regulates Bone Mass in Mice." *Journal of Bone and Mineral Research* 27, no. 6 (June 2012): 1357–1367. doi:10.1002/jbmr.1588.

Sowers, M. F., J. L. Beebe, D. McConnell, John Randolph, and M. Jannausch. "Testosterone Concentrations in Women Aged 25–50 Years: Associations with Lifestyle, Body Composition, and Ovarian Status." *American Journal of Epidemiology* 153, no. 3 (2001): 256–264.

Stenblom, Eva-Lena, Caroline Montelius, Karolina Östbring, Maria Håkansson, Sofia Nilsson, Jens F. Rehfeld, and Charlotte Erlanson-Albertsson. "Supplementation by thylakoids to a high carbohydrate meal decreases feelings of hunger, elevates CCK levels and prevents postprandial hypoglycaemia in overweight women." *Appetite* 68 (2013): 118–123. doi:10.1016/j.appet.2013.04.022.

Stenblom, Eva-Lena, Emil Egecioglu, Mona Landin-Olsson, and Charlotte Erlanson-Albertsson. "Consumption of thylakoid-rich spinach extract reduces hunger, increases satiety and reduces cravings for palatable food in overweight women." *Appetite* 91 (2015): 209–219. doi:10.1016/j.appet.2015.04.051.

Suez, Jotham, Tal Korem, David Zeevi, Gili Zilberman-Schapira, Christoph A. Thaiss, Ori Maza, David Israeli et al. "Artificial sweeteners induce glucose intolerance by altering the gut microbiota." *Nature* 514 (9 October 2014):181–186. doi:10.1038/nature13793.

Sze, Marc A., James C. Hogg, and Don D. Sin. "Bacterial microbiome of lungs in COPD." *International Journal of COPD* 9 (2014): 229–238. doi:10.2147/COPD.S38932.

Tai, Ningwen, F. Susan Wong, and Li Wen. "The role of gut microbiota in the development of type 1, obesity and type 2 diabetes mellitus." *Rev Endocr Metab Disord* 16, no. 1 (March 2015): 55–65. doi:10.1007/s11154-015-9309-0.

Talaei, Mohammad, and An Pan. "Role of phytoestrogens in prevention and management of type 2 diabetes." *World Journal of Diabetes* 6, no. 2 (2015): 271–283. doi:10.4239/wjd.v6.i2.271.

Taverniti, Valentina, and Simone Guglielmetti. "Health-promoting properties of Lactobacillus helveticus." *Frontiers in Microbiology* (2012). doi:10.3389/fmicb.2012.00392.

Wu, Gary D., Charlene Compher, Eric Z. Chen, Sarah A. Smith, Rachana D. Shah, Kyle Bittinger, Christel Chehoud et al. "Comparative metabolomics in vegans and omnivores reveal constraints on diet-dependent gut microbiota metabolite production." *Gut* 65, no. 1 (January 2016): 63–72. doi:10.1136/gutjnl-2014-308209.

Yamamoto, Mayuko, and Satoshi Matsumoto. "Gut microbiota and colorectal cancer." *Genes and Environment* 38, no. 11 (2016). doi:10.1186/s41021-016-0038-8.

Yurkovetskiy, Leonid, Michael Burrows, Aly A. Khan, Laura Graham, Pavel Volchkov, Lev Becker, Dionysios Antonopoulos, Yoshinori Umesaki, and Alexander V. Chervonsky. "Gender bias in autoimmunity is influenced by microbiota." *Immunity* 39, no. 2 (August 2013). doi:10.1016/j.immuni.2013.08.013.

Zhu, Yingying, Xisha Lin, He Li, Yingqiu Li, Xuebin Shi, Fan Zhao, Xinglian Xu, Chunbao Li, and Guanghong Zhou. "Intake of Meat Proteins Substantially Increased the Relative Abundance of Genus Lactobacillus in Rat Feces." *PLOS ONE* 11, no. 4 (2016). doi:10.1371/journal.pone.0152678.

CHAPTER 6

Barron, Anna M., and Christian J. Pike. "Sex hormones, aging, and Alzheimer's disease." *Frontiers in Bioscience* 4 (January 2012): 976–997.

Davis, Andra S., Kay Gilbert, Philip Misiowiec, and Barbara Riegel. "Perceived Effects of Testosterone Replacement Therapy in Perimenopausal and Postmenopausal Women: an Internet Pilot Study." *Health Care for Women International* 24 (2003): 831–848. doi: 10 1080/07399330390229902.

Davis, Susan R., Fiona Jane, Penelope J. Rbinson, Sonia L. Davison, Roisin Worsley, Paul Maruff, and Robin J. Bell.

"Transdermal testosterone improves verbal learning and memory in postmenopausal women not on oestrogen therapy." *Clinical Endocrinology* 81 (2014): 641–628. doi: 10.1111/cen.12459.

Davis, Susan R., Sarah Wahlin-Jacobsen. "Testosterone in women— the clinical significance." T*he Lancet Diabetes & Endocrinology* 3 (2015): 980–992.

Doty, Richard L., Isabelle Tourbier, Victoria Ng, Jessica Neff, Deborah Armstrong, Michelle Battistini, Mary D. Sammel et al. "Influences of Hormone Replacement Therapy on Olfactory and Cognitive Function in the Menopause." *Neurobiol Aging* 36, no. 6 (June 2015): 2053–2059. doi:10.1016/j.neurobiolaging.2015.02.028.

Glaser, Rebecca L., Mark Newman, Melanie Parsons, David Zava, and Daniel Glaser-Garbrick. "Safety of Maternal Testosterone Therapy during Breast Feeding." *International Journal of Pharmaceutical Compounding* 13, no. 4 (July/August 2009): 314–317.

Glaser, Rebecca, Constantine Dimitrakakis, Nancy Trimble, and Vincent Martin. "Testosterone pellet implants and migraine headaches: A pilot study." *Maturitas* 71, no. 4 (April 2012): 385–388. doi: 10.1016/j.maturitas.2012.01.006.

Gold, Stefan M. and Rhonda R. Voskuhl. "Estrogen Treatment in Multiple Sclerosis." *Journal of the Neurological Sciences*

286, no. 1–2 (November 2009): 99–103. doi:10.1016/j. jns.2009.05.028.

Gold, Stefan M. and Rhonda R. Voskuhl. "Estrogen and Testosterone Therapies in Multiple Sclerosis." *Progress in Brain Research* 175 (2009): 239–251. doi:10.1016/S0079-6123(09)17516-7.

Goldstat, Rebecca, Esther Briganti, Jane Tran, Rory Wolfe, and Susan R. Davis. "Transdermal testosterone therapy improves well-being, mood, and sexual function in premenopausal women." *Menopause: The Journal of The North American Menopause Society* 10, no. 5 (2003): 390–398. doi: 10.1097/ OI.GME.0000060256.03945.20.

Floter, A., J. Nathorst-Böös, K. Carlström, and B. von Schoultz. "Addition of testosterone to estrogen replacement therapy in oophorectomized women: effects on sexuality and well-being." *Climacteric* 5 (2002): 357–365.

Jovanovic, Hristina, Ljiljana Kocoska-Maras, Angelique Flöter Rådestad, Christer Halldina, Jacqueline Borg, Angelica Lindén Hirschberg, and Anna-Lena Nordström. "Effects of estrogen and testosterone treatment on serotonin transporter binding in the brain of surgically postmenopausal women – a PET study." *NeuroImage* 106 (2015): 47–54.

Maki, Pauline M. and Victor W. Henderson. "Hormone therapy, dementia, and cognition: the Women's Health Initiative ten years on." *Climacteric* 15, no. 3 (June 2012): 256–262. doi:10 .3109/13697137.2012.660613.

O'Brien, Jacqueline, John W. Jackson, Francine Grodstein, Deborah Blacker, and Jennifer Weuve. "Postmenopausal Hormone Therapy Is Not Associated with Risk of All-Cause Dementia and Alzheimer's Disease." *Epidemiologic Reviews* 36 (2014): 83–103. doi: 10.1093/epirev/mxt008.

Pike, Christian J., Jenna C. Carroll, Emily R. Rosario, and Anna M. Barron. "Protective actions of sex steroid hormones in Alzheimer's disease." *Frontiers in Neuroendocrinology* 30 (2009): 239–258. doi:10.1016/j.yfrne.2009.04.015.

Postma, Albert, Ghislaine Meyer, Adriaan Tuiten, Jack van Honk, Roy P.C. Kessels, and Jos Thijssen. "Effects of testosterone administration on selective aspects of object-location memory in healthy young women." *Psychoneuroendocrinology* 25 (2000): 563–575.

Rasgon, Natalie L., Cheri L. Geist, Heather A. Kenna, Tonita E. Wroolie, Katherine E. Williams, and Daniel H.S. Silverman. "Prospective Randomized Trial to Assess Effects of Continuing Hormone Therapy on Cerebral Function in Postmenopausal Women at Risk for Dementia." *PLOS ONE* 9, no. 3 (2014). doi:10.1371/journal.pone.0089095.

Ryan, J. J. Scali, I. Carriere, H. Amieva, O. Rouaud, C. Berr, K. Ritchie, and M-L. Ancelin. "Impact of a premature menopause on cognitive function in later life." BJOG: *An International Journal of Obstetrics & Gynaecology* 121, no. 13 (December 2014): 1729–1739. doi: 10.1111/1471-0528.12828.

Sicotte, Nancy L., Stephanie M. Liva, Rochelle Klutch, Paul Pfeiffer, Seth Bouvier, Sylvia Odesa, T. C. Jackson, and Rhonda R. Voskuhl. "Treatment of multiple sclerosis with the pregnancy hormone estriol." *Annals of Neurology* 52, no. 4 (August 2002): 421–428. doi: 10.1002/ana.10301.

Studd, John. "Hormone therapy for reproductive depression in women." *Post Reproductive Health* 20, no. 4 (2014): 132–137. doi: 10.1177/2053369114557883.

Voskuhl, Rhonda R., HeJing Wang, T. C. Jackson Wu, Nancy L. Sicotte, Kunio Nakamura, Florian Kurth, Noriko Itoh et al. "Estriol combined with glatiramer acetate for women with relapsing-remitting multiple sclerosis: a randomized, placebo-controlled, phase 2 trial." *Lancet Neural* 15 (2016): 35–46.

Xu, Jing, Lei-Lei Xia, Ning Song, Sheng-Di Chen, and Gang Wang. "Tesosterone, Estradiol, and Sex Hormone-Binding Globulin in Alzheimer's Disease: A Meta-Analysis." *Current Alzheimer Research* 13 (2016): 215–222.

Zandi, Peter P., Michelle C. Carlson, Brenda L. Plassman, Kathleen A. Welsh-Bohmer, Lawrence S. Mayer, David C. Steffens, John C. S. Breitner. "Hormone Replacement Therapy and Incidence of Alzheimer Disease in Older Women." *Journal of the American Medical Association* 288, no. 17 (November 2002): 2123–2129.

CHAPTER 7

Comhaire, F. "Hormone replacement therapy and longevity." *Andrologia* 48 (2016): 65–68. doi: 10.1111/and.12419.

Glaser, R. L., C. Dimitrakakis, and A. G. Messenger. "Improvement in scalp hair growth in androgen-deficient women treated with testosterone: a questionnaire study." *British Journal of Dermatology* 166 (2012): 274–278. doi: 10.1111/j.1365-2133.2011.10655.x.

Hall, Glenda and Tania J. Phillips. "Estrogen and skin: The effects of estrogen, menopause, and hormone replacement therapy on the skin." *Journal of the American Academy of Dermatology* 53, no. 4 (October 2005): 555–568. doi:10.1016/j.jaad.2004.08.039.

Horstman, Astrid M., E. Lichar Dillon, Randall J. Urban, and Melinda Sheffield-Moore. "The Role of Androgens and Estrogens on Healthy Aging and Longevity." *Journals of Gerontology* 67, no. 11 (November 2012): 1140–1152. doi:10.1093/gerona/gls068.

Kainz, C. G. Gitsch, J. Stani, G. Breitenecker, M. Binder, and J. B. Schmidt. "When applied to facial skin, does estrogen ointment have systemic effects?" *Archives of Gynecology and Obstetrics* 253 (1993): 71–74.

Samaras, Nikolaos, Maria-Aikaterini Papadopoulou, Dimitrios Samaras, and Filippo Ongaro. "Off-label use of hormones as an antiaging strategy: a review." *Clinical Interventions in Aging* 9 (2014): 1175–1186.

Schmidt, Jolanta B., Martina Binder, Gabrielle Demschik, Christian Bieglmayer, and Angelika Reiner. "Treatment of Skin Aging with Topical Estrogens." *International Journal of Dermatology* 35, no. 9 (September 1996): 669–674.

Schmidt, J. B., M. Binder, W. Macheiner, Ch. Kainz, G. Gitsch, and Ch. Bieglmayer. "Treatment of skin ageing symptoms in perimenopausal females with estrogen compounds. A pilot study." *Maturitas* 20 (1994): 25–30.

Stevenson, Susan and Julie Thornton. "Effect of estrogens on skin aging and the potential role of SERMs." *Clinical Interventions in Aging* 2, no. 3 (2007): 283–297.

CONCLUSION

Burger, H. G., J. Hailes, M. Menlaus, J. Nelson, B. Hudson, and N. Balazs. "The management of persistent menopausal symptoms with oestradiol-testosterone implants: clinical, lipid and hormonal results." *Maturitas* 6 (1984): 351–358.

Glaser, Rebecca, Sophia Kalantaridou, and Constantine Dimitrakakis. "Testosterone implants in women: Pharmacological dosing for a physiologic effect." *Maturitas* 74 (2013): 179-184. doi:10.1016/j.maturitas.2012.11.004.

Slater, Cristin C., Howard N. Hodis, Wendy J. Mack, Donna Shoupe, Richard J. Paulson, and Frank Z. Stanczyk. "Markedly elevated levels of estrone sulfate after long-term oral, but not transdermal, administration of estradiol in postmenopausal women." *Menopause* 8, no. 3 (2001): 200–203.

Stanczyk, Frank Z., Donna Shoupe, Victoria Nunes, Priscilla Macias-Gonzales, Marcela A. Vijod, and Rogerio Lobo. "A randomized comparison of nonoral estradiol delivery in postmenopausal women." *Am J Ostret Gynecol* 159, no. 6 (December 1988): 1540–1546.